Independent Living Support

Independent Living Support

VISION LOSS RESOURCES IN ALL STATES INCLUDING GUAM, PUERTO RICO AND THE VIRGIN ISLANDS

Patrick J. Fischer

ISBN-13: 9780692839157 (Accessibility dot Net, Inc.)
ISBN-10: 0692839151

Contents

Introduction

THIS BOOK WAS WRITTEN TO help people with low vision and also to help those who are trying to help someone else with low vision. This is a simple book and one that can be used as a resource guide.

If you have low vision, you are not alone. According to the National Eye Institute, millions of Americans and about 135 million people worldwide have low vision. Having worked with technology in the blind and visually impaired field since 1990, I know this book is needed today. This book will give you some basic information about eye doctors, low vision, low-vision aids, and the great low-vision-support options in your state. I will describe the low-cost technology aids that can help you now and let you know where you can find them. Lastly, this book will provide you with contact information for the best organizations in your own state that can help you now.

In 1985, I was sitting with my grandfather Francis, who had low vision and struggled with reading. He used a lighted magnifier with a 1.25-inch-square acrylic lens, which did help him read, although it was a very slow process. Grandpa told me that day that reading was very important to him; all his life, he had read in order to learn new things and keep up with what was going on in his community. The importance of reading cannot be overstated—it allows us to learn, grow, worship, and imagine. Reading is fundamentally a part of healthy living, and that is why I believe it is so crucial to help those with low vision retain the ability to read.

First and foremost (and you will hear me say this many times in this book), it is very important to get your eyes checked on a regular basis. Everyone needs to develop a relationship with an eye doctor in his or her community and get his or her eyes checked on a regular basis. All people at all ages need to get their eyes checked to ensure they have healthy eyes. Eye doctors can find the beginning stages of low vision, which will allow them to help you now and will prevent your vision from getting worse. If you have low vision, then an eye doctor who specializes in low vision can provide the best solutions to help you. The most important point I want to make in this book is to *get your eyes checked* on a regular basis!

In addition to encouraging you to see your eye doctor regularly, I also want to promote the low-cost solutions and great services available that can help you remain independent and allow you to read printed material. This book will explain what low vision is, introduce the low-cost technology aids that are available, and offer you a way to get help locally. This book will also help a person with low vision regain his or her self-confidence by providing ways to accomplish daily activities, remain independent, and continue to read.

What Is Good Vision?

To understand low vision, let's review what good vision is and how it works. Central vision is the vision we use when we look directly at something. It provides us the most detail to read print, thread a needle, and recognize faces. Peripheral vision is the vision we use around the edges of our central vision, and although it is not as detailed as central vision, it allows us to see a large visual field. When you hear someone say "I saw that out of the corner of my eye," that person is referring to using his or her peripheral vision.

What Is Low Vision?

Low vision is defined as visual impairments that are not correctable through surgery or corrected lenses. Low vision causes a reduction in visual acuity, visual field, or both. The term *low vision* is often used interchangeably with *visual impairment*. Low vision refers to a loss of vision that may be severe enough to prevent someone from completing daily activities such as reading, cooking, using a computer, or walking outside safely. With the proper help, a person with low vision can learn to complete his or her daily activities and live independently.

What Is Visual Acuity?

Visual acuity refers to the clarity and sharpness of vision. Visual acuity is measured by the ability to tell the difference between letters or numbers at a given distance according to a fixed standard. The visual acuity is the clinical measure of an eye and is usually given in a fraction to measure print size. This fraction refers to the clarity or sharpness of your vision. Normal visual acuity measured at a distance of twenty feet is expressed as 20/20 vision. If you have 20/20 vision, at twenty feet you can see clearly what should normally be seen at that distance. If an individual sees 20/200, the smallest letter that this individual can see at twenty feet could be seen by someone with 20/20 vision at two hundred feet.

Nearly two centuries ago, doctors agreed upon the standards of measurement of visual acuity (clarity and sharpness) that define "normal" vision for people. The familiar chart that is still used by eye doctors today to measure visual acuity is called Snellen's Chart.

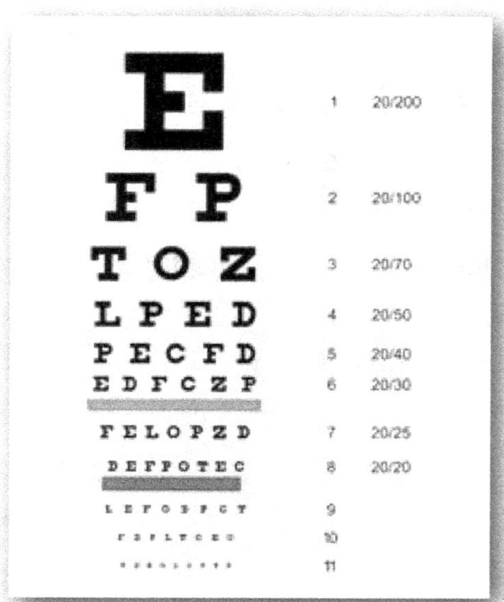

Snellen's Chart was invented by a Dutch ophthalmologist named Hermann Snellen (1834–1908). Even the specialized lettering used on the chart was developed by Dr. Snellen, and this type of lettering remains the same today. Dr. Snellen, along with some of his colleagues, found that twenty feet is the distance at which the average, healthy eye is able to see clearly without strain or compensation.

What Is Visual Field?

Visual field refers to the total area in which objects can be seen in the side (peripheral) vision as you focus your eyes on a central point. The visual field is the total area seen while looking straight ahead without moving your eyes.

What Is Blindness?

Legal blindness is a level of vision loss that has been legally defined to determine eligibility for benefits. The clinical diagnosis for legal blindness refers to a central visual acuity of 20/200 or less in the better eye with the best possible correction and/or a visual field of twenty degrees or less. Many people who are diagnosed with legal blindness still have some useable vision. Total blindness refers to an inability to see anything with either eye.

Eye Doctors and Vision Professionals

THERE ARE TWO TYPES OF eye doctors: optometrists and ophthalmologists. There are also other important professionals in an eye doctor's office, including opticians, assistive-technology specialist, orientation and mobility specialists, occupational therapists, and vision-rehabilitation therapists.

OPTOMETRISTS

An optometrist is an eye doctor who has earned a Doctor of Optometry (OD) degree. Optometrists examine eyes for both vision and health problems and correct refractive errors by prescribing eyeglasses and contact lenses. They often have someone on their staff to provide low-vision care and vision therapy, or they can refer you to a low-vision specialist in your area. Later in the book, I list out a link in your state so you can find an optometrist in your area.

Ophthalmologists

An ophthalmologist is a medical doctor (MD) who specializes in eye and vision care. Ophthalmologists are trained to perform the full spectrum of eye care, including conducting exams, diagnosing and treating disease, prescribing medications, and performing specialized eye surgery. They also write prescriptions for eyeglasses and contact lenses. They often have someone on their staff to provide low-vision care and vision therapy, or they can refer you to a low-vision specialist in your area. Later in the book, I list out a link in your state so you can find an ophthalmologist in your area.

Opticians

An optician uses prescriptions written by an ophthalmologist or an optometrist to properly fit and sell eyeglasses and other eyewear for patients.

Other Specialists

Low-vision rehabilitation is a service provided by a team made up of a assistive-technology specialists, orientation and mobility specialists, occupational therapists, vision-rehabilitation therapists, and other professionals. Low-vision rehabilitation services allow people who are blind or have low vision to continue to live independently and maintain quality of life.

An assistive-technology specialist is an individual who provides products and services that are designed to assist people with disabilities to choose, acquire, or use assistive-technology devices.

An orientation and mobility (O and M) specialist can help a person with low vision learn to move about safely in his or her home and travel outside without assistance.

Occupational therapists are professionals who help people remain independent. Some specialize in low-vision rehabilitation and can train people with low vision to use magnifiers, talking devices, and other assistive-technology aids. They can provide treatment only with the prescription of a medical doctor or a doctor of optometry.

Vision-rehabilitation therapists are specialists in independent living who train people with low vision to perform a wide range of daily activities.

Common Types of Visual Impairment

THE PICTURE BELOW SHOWS FOUR children as seen with 20/20 (normal) vision.

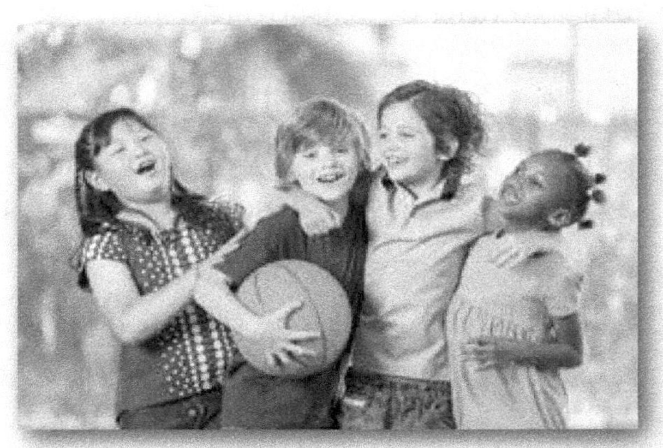

Below are four pictures that have been altered from the first picture to give you an idea of how vision is affected by the most common types of visual impairments. These altered pictures are based on other pictures available to the public that show the same comparison.

The most common types of visual impairment are

- cataract;
- glaucoma;
- retinitis pigmentosa (RP); and
- age-related macular degeneration (AMD).

<table>
<tr>
<td>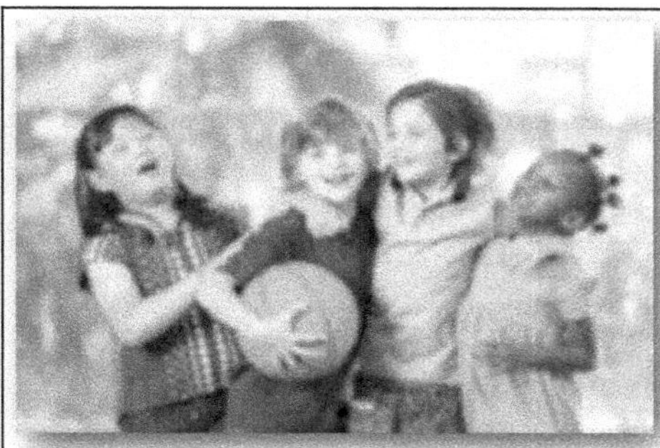</td>
<td>Cataract is a clouding of the lens of the eye and causes vision to be blurry. Cataracts are the leading cause of visual impairment in the world.

It is important to see your eye doctor for regular eye examinations. Cataract surgery is generally very successful in restoring vision. In fact, it is the most frequently performed eye surgery in the United States.</td>
</tr>
</table>

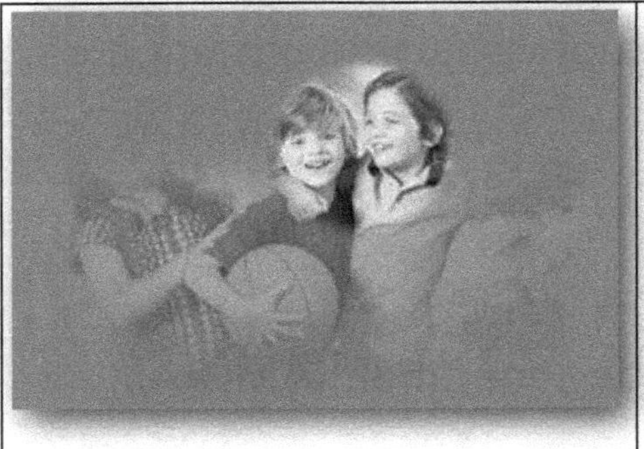	Glaucoma is a complicated disease that leads to progressive, irreversible vision loss. It is important to see your eye doctor for regular eye examinations. If glaucoma is detected during an eye exam, your eye doctor can prescribe a preventative treatment to help protect your vision.
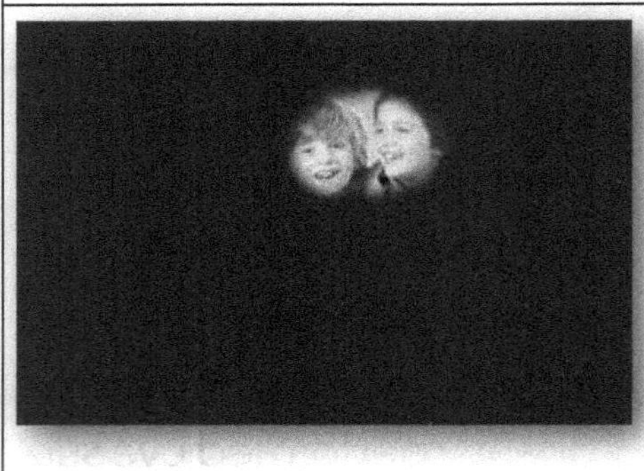	Retinitis pigmentosa (RP) may appear at any age, but it usually begins in childhood or adolescence. At first, the person has trouble seeing in dim light. The visual field gradually narrows, causing tunnel vision. Tunnel vision looks like you are looking through a tube.

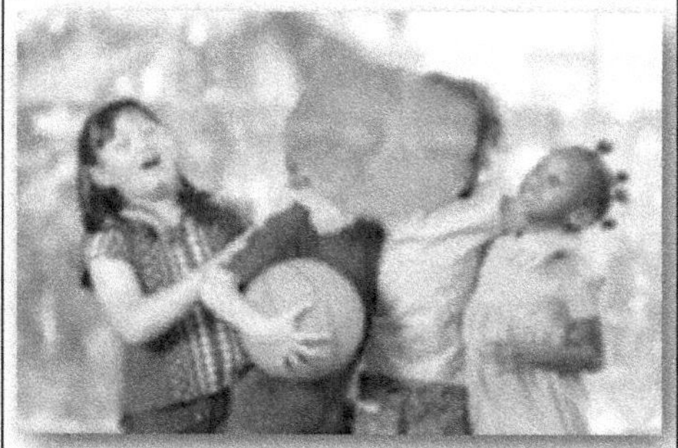	Age-Related Macular Degeneration (AMD) is the leading cause of vision loss in the United States. Macular degeneration gradually affects central vision, and the person may experience blurred, distorted, or dim vision. It is very important for people with macular degeneration to monitor their eyesight carefully and see their eye doctor on a regular basis.

Additional causes of low vision include strokes, diabetic retinopathy, traumatic brain injury (TBI), and other diseases, such as Stargardt's, and retinopathy of prematurity (ROP).

Low-Vision Aids

As you learn about people with low vision, you will understand that even if two people have the same type of low vision, different low-vision aids might help them. It is important to try different solutions until you find what best helps you. While one person may choose to read large print, others will use magnification, and still others will learn to use braille. Some people may have difficulty recognizing faces but may be able to read standard print with special glasses. When it comes to low vision, at one end there are various degrees of low vision and at the other end is blindness.

Low-vision aids break into several categories, and while some people may need to use items in all of the categories of low-vision aids, other people may only use a few items in a few categories. An important point to remember is that everyone is different and therefore has different needs, so you may have to try a lot of products until you find what works best for you.

There are many options for visual aids; to make it easy to learn, I have divided the most common visual aids into the following categories: contrast, lighting, tactile markings, talking gadgets, large print, and over-the-counter magnifiers.

Since the majority of our time is spent at home, the first area to talk about making changes will be the home. These changes can also be made at your job with your employer's assistance. Two of the easiest areas to change are contrast and lighting. Always compare different choices so you can find what best helps you or the person you are helping.

Contrast

When you modify your environment to make it more accessible for you or the person with low vision, contrast is very important to keep in mind. Contrast is defined as two things that are very different from each other—for example, making this **text bold** gives it great contrast compared to the other text.

Take the colors black and white as an example. These two colors are the opposite of each other. Black and white next to each other are the best example of contrast.

The person with low vision will let you know what colors he or she can see best, so make sure to display the different colors so that he or she can choose the best contrast. If you go to a paint store, you can pick up paint chips of different colors to look at or show the person with low vision you are helping. Keep in mind that colors are divided into two categories: warm and cool, which contrast with each other. Cool colors are blue, green, and purple; they give the impression of calmness and cooler temperatures. Warm colors are yellow, orange, and red and are vivid and associated with warmer temperatures.

Changing colors to make a good contrast is an easy example that can really help a person with low vision. As an example, if your kitchen table is white, then dark-colored dishes offer the best contrast. This is an easy one to solve, as you can get a tablecloth that is the opposite color of your dishes.

Having the proper contrast in your home or office can make life more pleasant for a person with low vision, because he or she will easily be able to see what is needed to function.

Areas where you want to have proper contrast are where walls and floors meet, making it easier to walk from room to room. Stairs should have contrast on the steps so a person can see the edge of each step. Putting a strip of colored tape on the edge of each stair provides great contrast. Every path you take in your home, along with every room you use, should be looked at and modified for the proper contrast.

You can look inside every drawer in your home and make the necessary changes so it will be easier to see what you are looking for. Change the colors of the inside of a drawer or maybe even get utensils that have colored handles so that the contrast will help you see what you need. Do whatever you have to do to make it easier to see and find what you are looking for. Reduce clutter and get rid of items not used so that it is easy to find what you need. Make your home and office the most organized you can and create contrast so that everything stands out and can be seen. These are simple changes to make, and they make a huge difference to the person with low vision.

Making these simple modifications to your environment will make it easy to walk around and find things as you need them. With the proper contrast, a person with low vision will be empowered and feel better at home or at work.

Lighting

Lighting is an inexpensive solution that can greatly help a person with low vision read and remain independent. It is very important for safety reasons because it can help prevent accidents. Remember that everyone is different and someone with low vision generally needs more than one light source in a room, although some people may need less light.

Sunlight is a great light source but one that you need to control. Having blinds on a window are great because they allow a person to let light in and close light out as needed. Having the window blinds turned so the sunlight shines upward is best for some people, although sometimes you may want the window blinds turned so the sunlight shines downward.

Placing table and floor lamps next to the tables and chairs where reading takes place is also very important. Extra lights in halls and closets can help too. How you turn lights on is also very important. Pull strings are generally no fun to use because the string can be hard to see. A light switch that is always in the same place is best.

Always remember, what works for one person in terms of lighting may not work for another person. The best way to figure out what you need is to try different lights and experiment to find out what works best for you. You will be so happy once you improve your contrast and lighting!

Visit the Low Vision Support website (LowVisionSupport.com) for some lighting products.

Tactile Markings

Tactile markings are inexpensive items such as bump dots, puff paint, or even small pieces of felt. We place tactile markings to help a person with low vision identify important settings and buttons on appliances, which makes it easier for the person to use these items. Tactile markings can be applied to stoves, microwaves, washers, dryers, telephones, and other appliances where you need to push a button or turn a dial to a certain point. Remember the importance of contrast as you purchase tactile markings, because they come in different colors. Always purchase tactile markings that provide the proper contrast for the person with low vision so he or she can see the tactile markings—use dark markings on a light background and light markings on a dark background. A low-vision specialist can help you discover the best approach to these situations.

Placing tactile markings on the outside of a dial helps a person with low vision feel for the proper place to stop when turning the dial. With the help of a low-vision specialist, these can be applied to the proper location so the person with low vision will not rely on trying to see it but instead will feel for the proper place to set a control. Stoves with digital displays are a little tricky, but a magnifier can be used to help those with low vision see settings like setting the oven temperature. Over-the-counter magnifiers will be discussed later in this book.

Puff paint is a great product to add tactile markings to almost anything, including paper, wood, cloth, and metal. It is a craft material used to add both texture and a great look and feel to an item. Unlike other paints that have a two-dimensional look, puff paint has a raised, three-dimensional appearance, which is great for persons with low vision. Puff paint is versatile because it adheres well to different surfaces. Apply puff paint directly from its tube applicator onto areas that you need to feel a tactile marking. A great place to use puff paint is a cable that has a top and bottom. A person with low vision can usually not see what is the top or the bottom because the markings are small; a small spot of puff paint on one side makes it easy to use. Another great benefit to puff paint is that it comes in multiple colors, which helps with creating contrast.

Puff paint is my favorite tactile marking product because it adds a three-dimensional raised marking and comes in different colors, which makes a perfect solution for persons with low vision. Puff paint dries in approximately two to four hours, depending on the surface and thickness of marks. You can purchase individual tubes in common colors of red, yellow, blue, green, white, and black.

Visit the Low Vision Support website (LowVisionSupport.com) for some Tactile products

Talking Gadgets

Talking gadgets are electronics that speak the information you would normally read with your eyes. These devices are very helpful for someone with low vision, because rather than strain to see something, all you have to do is press a button. There are many different types of talking gadgets. The following are the most common items used by those with low vision:

- clocks
- health products, including blood glucose monitors, thermometers, and blood pressure readers

- calculators
- scales

Visit the Low Vision Support website (LowVisionSupport.com) for some talking gadget products.

Large Print

Large print refers to the formatting of a book or other text document in which the font is considerably larger than usual, to accommodate people who have low vision. Sixteen point or higher type is considered the industry standard for large print.

The most popular large print items are large print calendars, address books, and check registers. The Jumbo Large Print Calendar is the most popular product in the large print family because it is useful for everyone. The Jumbo Large Print Calendar measures twenty-two by seventeen inches and comes ready for wall mounting. This handy calendar is made of white heavy bond paper with bold black print and a plastic spiral, making it easy to change months. There is plenty of room on each day and each calendar page for notes and appointments.

Large print books are a whole category, and many books are available. Amazon.com has the largest selection of large print books available for purchase, and finding books is easy because they are broken out into categories. These books are unabridged and contain the original content; they are not condensed or shortened in any way. If you read a book on a Kindle or other tablet, then you can increase the size of the font and make every book large print.

For persons who are legally blind, there is a national network of cooperating libraries, the National Library Service (NLS) which is a free library program of audiobooks and materials that are circulated by postage-free mail. In addition, BARD (Braille and Audio Reading Download) Mobile can be used to access talking books on various devices (versions are available for iOS, Android, and Kindle). Later in the book, I list out all of the library's in your state so you can sign up for the NLS and BARD library program.

Visit the Low Vision Support website (LowVisionSupport.com) for some large print products.

Over-the-Counter Magnifiers

Over-the-counter magnifiers are useful for those with low vision. Some magnifiers have a light, and some do not. Some inexpensive magnifiers are made of hard plastic, and I do not recommend these because they typically have a limited magnification power and are easy to scratch. Bright, illuminated, handheld LED optic magnifiers are the best with magnification levels starting at 2X and going up to 5X and much higher. These can be purchased for between sixty and one hundred dollars. These can be easily carried in a purse or pocket. A magnifier with a large diameter typically offers more viewing area but less power. The greater the magnification, the smaller the lens.

When you have an appliance in your home or office that uses an LCD to display information, then an optic magnifier can be a great tool to use to see the display. Depending on the LCD display, it may work better to use the light on your magnifying device, and it may not. You should try both options to see which works best.

Dome magnifiers are dome-shaped and are easy to use. Many people with low vision find they are great for reading newspapers, mail, and other printed materials. To use, you glide the dome magnifier over the material you are reading. These magnifiers also make great paperweights when you are not using them.

Visit the Low Vision Support website (LowVisionSupport.com) for see some over-the-counter and dome magnifiers products.

Directory of Services and Resources

UP TO THIS POINT, YOU have learned about many things that can help you with low vision—or can help the person with low vision you are assisting. To close out this book, I will provide a state-by-state list of the most important organizations to contact if you need local assistance. I promise you—these organizations can help you.

- **State Agency for the Blind and Visually Impaired**
  Find resources and support for families and friends of people with low vision. Contact your state agency and learn about the local help they can provide you now.
- **State Office—Veterans Affairs - Visual Impairment Services Team (VIST)**
  The VA Visual Impairment Services Team program provides services to veterans and active duty service members experiencing vision loss. Veterans contact your local VIST Coordinator and get local help now.

- **American Optometric Association**
  Doctors of Optometry provide two thirds of all primary eye care in the United States. Use this site to find an optometrist in your area.
- **American Academy of Ophthalmology**
  This is the world's largest association of eye physicians and surgeons. Use this site to find an ophthalmologist in your area.
- **NEI's National Eye Health Education Program (NEHEP)**
  The National Eye Institute (NEI) established the National Eye Health Education Program (NEHEP) to help health and community professionals increase awareness about eye health. NEHEP programs promote the use of vision rehabilitation services.
- **State Organizations and Businesses Providing Low-Vision Support, Products, and Services**
  This is a list of organizations that help persons with low vision. I personally know many on this list, and the others come highly recommended.
- **Lions Clubs International**
  In 1925 Helen Keller challenged the Lions to be "knights of the blind in the crusade against darkness." Since then, Lions have dedicated themselves to preventing blindness, restoring sight, and improving eye care services. The Lions are

the world's largest service club organization, and their members do whatever is needed to help their local communities. Use this site to find a lions club in your area.

- **State Office for National Library Services (NLS)** Through a national network of cooperating libraries, NLS administers a free library program of audio books and materials. Find the library in your state, so you can sign up for the NLS library program and get free books to read.

Directory

ALABAMA

State Agency for the Blind and Visually Impaired

Alabama Department of Rehabilitation Services
602 S. Lawrence Street
Montgomery, AL 36104
334-293-7500
http://www.rehab.alabama.gov

State Office—VA Visual Impairment Services Team (VIST)

VA Medical Center
700 S. Nineteenth Street
Birmingham, AL 35233
205-933-4389

Central Alabama Veterans Health Care System
East Campus 2400 Hospital Road
Tuskegee, AL 36083
334-727-0550 x3459

Tuscaloosa VAMC
3701 Loop Road, East
Tuscaloosa, AL 35404
205-554-3542

American Optometric Association
http://www.aoa.org/doctor-locator-search?tab=basic&sso=y

American Academy of Ophthalmology
https://secure.aao.org/aao/find-ophthalmologist

NEI's National Eye Health Education Program
https://nei.nih.gov/nehep

State Organizations and Businesses Providing Low-Vision Support, Products, and Services
Alabama UAB Center for Low Vision Rehabilitation
Callahan Eye Foundation Hospital
700 Eighteenth Street, Suite 405
South Birmingham, AL 35294
205-488-0736
https://www.uab.edu/medicine/ophthalmology/patient-care/clinical-services/clvr

Community Services for Vision Rehabilitation CSVR
600 BelAir Boulevard, Suite 110

Mobile, AL 36606
251-476-4744 in Mobile
251-928-2888 in Daphne
228-760-0788 in Gulfport
334-782-3557 in Montgomery
www.csvrlowvision.org

Lions Clubs International
https://directory.lionsclubs.org/?language=EN

State Office for National Library Services (NLS)
Alabama Regional Library for the Blind and Physically Handicapped
6030 Monticello Drive
Montgomery, AL 36130-6000
334-213-3921 or 334-213-3906
http://statelibrary.alabama.gov/Content/APLSSer_Blind.aspx
Serves: Alabama (63 of 67 counties)

Huntsville Subregional Library for the Blind and Physically Handicapped
PO Box 443
Huntsville, AL 35804-0000
256-532-5980
http://hmcpl.org/departments
Serves: Madison County

Library and Resource Center for the Blind and Physically Handicapped
Alabama Institute for Deaf and Blind
705 South Street E
PO Box 698
Talladega, AL 35161-0000
256-761-3237
http://www.aidb.org
Serves: Talladega, Calhoun, and St. Clair counties

ALASKA

State Agency for the Blind and Visually Impaired
Alaska Center for the Blind and Visually Impaired
3903 Taft Drive
Anchorage, AK 99517-3069
907-248-7770
http://www.alaskabvi.org/

State Office—VA Visual Impairment Services Team (VIST)
Alaska VA Healthcare System and Regional Office
2925 DeBarr Road
Anchorage, AK 99508-2989
907-257-3776

American Optometric Association
http://www.aoa.org/doctor-locator-search?tab=basic&sso=y

American Academy of Ophthalmology
https://secure.aao.org/aao/find-ophthalmologist

NEI's National Eye Health Education Program
https://nei.nih.gov/nehep

State Organizations and Businesses Providing Low-Vision Support, Products, and Services
Alaska BVI Low Vision Clinic
http://www.alaskabvi.org/Our%20Services/LV%20CLINIC/Pages/default.aspx

Accurate Vision Clinic
207 E Northern Lights Blvd, Suite 101
Anchorage, AK 99503
907-312-5321
http://accuratevisionclinic.com/

Lions Clubs International
https://directory.lionsclubs.org/?language=EN

State Office for National Library Services (NLS)
Alaska State Library Talking Book Center
395 Whittier Street
Juneau, AK 99801
907-465-1304 or 907-465-1315
http://talkingbooks.alaska.gov
Serves: Alaska; the Alaska State Library Talking Book Center processes applications for Alaska patrons. The Utah State Library Program for the Blind and Disabled provides library materials, BARD assistance, and machine lending services to Alaska patrons.

ARIZONA

State Agency for the Blind and Visually Impaired
Arizona Center for the Blind and Visually Impaired
3100 E. Roosevelt Street
Phoenix, AZ 85008
602-273-7411
http://www.acbvi.org

State Office—VA Visual Impairment Services Team (VIST)
Carl T. Hayden VAMC
650 E. Indian School Road
Phoenix, AZ 85012
602-277-5551 x17236

Northern Arizona VA HCS
500 N. Hwy 89
Prescott, AZ 86313
928-445-4860 x6849

Southern Arizona VA HCS
3601 South 6th Avenue
Tucson, AZ 85723
520-792-1450 x15608
520-792-1450 x14501
520-792-1450 x15632

American Optometric Association
http://www.aoa.org/doctor-locator-search?tab=basic&sso=y

American Academy of Ophthalmology
https://secure.aao.org/aao/find-ophthalmologist

NEI's National Eye Health Education Program
https://nei.nih.gov/nehep

State Organizations and Businesses Providing Low-Vision Support, Products, and Services
View Finder Low Vision Resource Center
1830 S. Alma School Road, #131

Mesa, AZ 85210
480-924-8755
http://www.viewfinderlowvision.com/

View Finder Low Vision Resource Center
10001 W. Bell Road, #115
Sun City, AZ 85351
623-583-2800
http://www.viewfinderlowvision.com/

Lions Clubs International
https://directory.lionsclubs.org/?language=EN

State Office for National Library Services (NLS)
Arizona State Braille and Talking Book Library
1030 N. Thirty-Second Street
Phoenix, AZ 85008-5108
602-255-5578
http://www.azlibrary.gov/talkingbooks
Serves: Arizona; braille readers receive service from Utah.

Arkansas

State Agency for the Blind and Visually Impaired
Arkansas Department of Human Services: Division of Services for the Blind

700 Main Street, Slot 101
Little Rock, AR 72203-3237
501-682-5463
http://humanservices.arkansas.gov/dsb/Pages/default.aspx

State Office—VA Visual Impairment Services Team (VIST)
Fayetteville VHSO
1100 N. College Avenue
Fayetteville, AR 72703
479-443-4301 x65364

Central Arkansas Veterans
HCS John L. McClellan Memorial Veterans Hospital
4300 West 7th Street
Little Rock, AR 72205-5484
501-257-5070

American Optometric Association
http://www.aoa.org/doctor-locator-search?tab=basic&sso=y

American Academy of Ophthalmology
https://secure.aao.org/aao/find-ophthalmologist

NEI's National Eye Health Education Program
https://nei.nih.gov/nehep

State Organizations and Businesses Providing Low-Vision Support, Products, and Services

NanoPac Inc.
4823 S. Sheridan Road, Suite 302
Tulsa, OK 74145
800-580-6086
http://www.nanopac.com/

Jones Eye Institute
University of Arkansas for Medical Sciences
4301 W. Markham Street
Little Rock, AR 72205
501-686-5822
http://eye.uams.edu/specialties/low-vision/

Arkansas Lighthouse for the Blind
6818 Murray Street
Little Rock, AR 72219
501-562-2222
https://ifbsolutions.org/about/locations/arkansas/

Lions Clubs International

https://directory.lionsclubs.org/?language=EN

State Office for National Library Services (NLS)

Arkansas Regional Library for the Blind and Physically Handicapped

900 W. Capitol Avenue, Suite 100
Little Rock, AR 72201-3108
501-682-1155
http://www.library.arkansas.gov/
Serves: Arkansas

CALIFORNIA

State Agency for the Blind and Visually Impaired

California Department of Rehabilitation: Blind Field Services Division
721 Capitol Mall
Sacramento, CA 95814
916-558-5480
http://www.dor.ca.gov/SSD/Blind-Field-Services.html

State Office—VA Visual Impairment Services Team (VIST)

VA Central California HCS
2615 E. Clinton Avenue
Fresno, CA 93703
559-225-6100, x5252

VA Northern California
H10535 Hospital Way
Mather, CA 95655
916-843-7053

VA Palo Alto Health Care System
3801 Miranda Avenue
Palo Alto, CA 94304
650-852-3431

San Francisco VAMC
4150 Clement Street
San Francisco, CA 94121
415-750-6604

VA Long Beach HCS
5901 E. Seventh Street
Long Beach, CA 90822
562-826-8000, x5696

VA Loma Linda Healthcare System
11201 Benton Street
Loma Linda, CA 92357
909-825-7084, x2748

VA San Diego Healthcare System
3350 La Jolla Village Drive
San Diego, CA 92161
858-552-8585

VA Greater Los Angeles Healthcare System (GLA)
11301 Wilshire Boulevard
Los Angeles, CA 90073
310-478-3711, x44780

VA Greater Los Angeles Healthcare System (GLA)
16111 Plummer Street
Sepulveda, CA 91343
213-253-5050 (WLA)
818-895-9387 (Sep)
310-413-0247 (BB)

American Optometric Association
http://www.aoa.org/doctor-locator-search?tab=basic&sso=y

American Academy of Ophthalmology
https://secure.aao.org/aao/find-ophthalmologist

NEI's National Eye Health Education Program
https://nei.nih.gov/nehep

State Organizations and Businesses Providing Low-Vision Support, Products, and Services
The Frank Stein and Paul S. May Center for Low Vision Rehabilitation at California Pacific Medical Center

Department of Ophthalmology
2340 Clay Street, Fifth Floor
San Francisco, CA 94115
415-600-3901
http://www.cpmc.org/services/eye/LVRprogram.html

Lighthouse for the Blind and Visually Impaired
Adaptations Store
1155 Market St., 10th Floor
San Francisco, CA 94103
415-431-1481
http://www.lighthouse-sf.org

Blind & Visually Impaired Center of Monterey County Inc.
225 Laurel Avenue
Pacific Grove, CA 93950
831-649-3505
http://www.blindandlowvision.org

Center for the Blind & Visually Impaired
1721 Westwind Drive, Suite B
Bakersfield, CA 93301
661-322-5234
http://www.cbvi.org

Center for the Partially Sighted
6101 W. Centinela Avenue, Suite 150
Culver City, CA 90030
310-988-1970
http://www.low-vision.org/services/optometric/

Lions Center for the Visually Impaired of Diablo Valley
175 Alvarado Avenue
Pittsburg, CA 94565
925-432-3013
http://seniorvision.org/

San Diego Center for the Blind and Vision Impaired
5922 El Cajon Boulevard
San Diego, CA 92115
619-583-1542
https://www.sdcb.org/SDCB-Store

Society for the Blind
1238 S Street
Sacramento, CA 95811
916-452-8271
http://societyfortheblind.org/low-vision-clinic/your-low-vision-evaluation/

St. Mary Low Vision Center
1055 Linden Avenue

Long Beach, CA 90813
562-491-9275
http://www.dignityhealth.org/stmarymedical/community-benefits/low-vision-center

The Smith-Kettlewell Eye Research Institute: Rehabilitation Engineering Research Center
2318 Fillmore Street
San Francisco, CA 94115
415-345-2110
http://www.ski.org/event-type/low-vision-support-group

Optometry Clinic
Beckman Vision Center
8 Koret Way
Suites U-545 and U519
San Francisco, CA 94143-0344
415-514-8200
https://www.ucsfhealth.org/clinics/optometry/

University of California: School of Optometry, Low Vision Clinic
200 Minor Hall
Berkeley, CA 94720-2020
510-642-5726
http://www.caleyecare.org/services/low-vision-exams

Vista Center, Palo Alto—Low Vision Clinic
3200 Hillview Avenue, Suite 120
Palo Alto, CA 94304
650-858-0202
http://www.vistacenter.org/low_vision_clinic.html

Vista Center, Santa Cruz—Low Vision Clinic
413 Laurel Street
Santa Cruz, CA 95060
831-458-9766
http://www.vistacenter.org

Watts Health Care Corporation
10300 Compton Avenue
Los Angeles, CA 90002
323-564-4331
http://www.wattshealth.org/clinical-services/vision-care/

Lions Clubs International
https://directory.lionsclubs.org/?language=EN

State Office for National Library Services (NLS)
Braille and Talking Book Library
California State Library
900 N Street

Sacramento, CA 95814-4811
916-654-0640
http://www.btbl.ca.gov
Serves: Alameda, Alpine, Amador, Butte, Calaveras, Colusa, Contra Costa, Del Norte, El Dorado, Fresno, Glen, Humboldt, Inyo, Kings, Lake, Lassen, Marin, Madera, Mariposa, Mendocino, Merced, Modoc, Mono, Monterey, Napa, Nevada, Placer, Plumas, Sacramento, San Benito, San Joaquin, San Mateo, Santa Clara, Santa Cruz, Shasta, Sierra, Siskiyou, Solano, Sonoma, Stanislaus, Sutter, Tehama, Trinity, Tulare, Tuolumne, Yolo, and Yuba; braille: Fresno, Kings, Madera, Tulare, and San Francisco

Braille Institute
Library Services
741 N. Vermont Avenue
Los Angeles, CA 90029-3594
323-660-3880
http://www.braillelibrary.org/
Serves: Imperial, Kern, Los Angeles, Orange, Riverside, San Bernardino, San Diego, San Luis Obispo, Santa Barbara, and Ventura counties

Talking Book Library for the Blind
Fresno County Public Library
Ted Wills Community Center
770 N. San Pablo Avenue

Fresno, CA 93728-3640
559-600-3217
http://www.fresnolibrary.org/tblb
Serves: Fresno, Kings, Madera, and Tulare counties

Library for the Blind and Print Disabled
San Francisco Public Library
Civic Center
100 Larkin Street
San Francisco, CA 94102-0000
415-557-4253
http://sfpl.org/index.php?pg=0200002301
Serves: San Francisco

Colorado

State Agency for the Blind and Visually Impaired
Colorado Vocational Rehabilitation
1575 Sherman Street, Fourth Floor
Denver, CO 80203
303-866-4150
Office Locations: http://www.dvrcolorado.com/locations.php

State Office—VA Visual Impairment Services Team (VIST)
VA Eastern Colorado Health Care System (ECHCS)
1055 Clermont Street

Denver, CO 80220
303-399-8020, x3040

Pueblo Community-Based Out-Patient Clinic
4776 Eagleridge Circle
Pueblo, CO 81008
719-584-5126

Grand Junction VAMC
2121 North Avenue
Grand Junction, CO 81501
970-263-5080

American Optometric Association
http://www.aoa.org/doctor-locator-search?tab=basic&sso=y

American Academy of Ophthalmology
https://secure.aao.org/aao/find-ophthalmologist

NEI's National Eye Health Education Program
https://nei.nih.gov/nehep

State Organizations and Businesses Providing Low-Vision Support, Products, and Services
University of Colorado Vision Rehabilitation Service
University of Colorado School of Medicine

Department of Ophthalmology
1675 Aurora Court, F731
Aurora, CO 80045
720-848-2020
http://www.Eyeinstitute.org

Ensight Skills Center for Visual Rehabilitation
1740 S. College Avenue
Fort Collins, CO 80525
970-407-9999
http://www.ensightskills.org/

Ensight Skills Center—Greeley
918 Thirteenth Street, Suite 4
Greeley, CO 80631
970-353-9417

Low Vision Services of Southern Colorado
5614 N. Union Boulevard
Colorado Springs, CO 80918
719-471-3200
http://www.lowvisionsoco.com/

NanoPac Inc.
4823 S. Sheridan Road, Suite 302
Tulsa, OK 74145

800-580-6086
http://www.nanopac.com/

Colorado Center for the Blind
2233 W. Shepperd Avenue
Littleton, CO 80120
303-778-1130
http://www.cocenter.org

Center for Independence
740 Gunnison Avenue
Grand Junction, CO 81501
970-241-0315
http://www.cfigj.org/programs/low-vision

Lions Clubs International
https://directory.lionsclubs.org/?language=EN

State Office for National Library Services (NLS)
Colorado Talking Book Library
180 Sheridan Boulevard
Denver, CO 80226-8101
303-727-9277
http://www.myctbl.org

Connecticut

State Agency for the Blind and Visually Impaired

Department of Rehabilitation Services—Bureau of Education & Services for the Blind
184 Windsor Avenue
Windsor, CT 06095
860-602-4000
http://www.ct.gov/besb

State Office—VA Visual Impairment Services Team (VIST)

VA Connecticut Healthcare System, West Haven Campus
950 Campbell Avenue
West Haven, CT 06516
203-932-5711, x3407

American Optometric Association

http://www.aoa.org/doctor-locator-search?tab=basic&sso=y

American Academy of Ophthalmology

https://secure.aao.org/aao/find-ophthalmologist

NEI's National Eye Health Education Program

https://nei.nih.gov/nehep

State Organizations and Businesses Providing Low-Vision Support, Products, and Services

Healthy Eyes Alliance
129 Church Street, Suite 820

New Haven, CT 06510
203-772-4652
www.healthyeyesalliance.org

Lions Low Vision Center of Eastern Connecticut
PO Box 43
Colchester, CT 06415
860-377-2063
http://www.lionslowvisionctr.org

Oak Hill
120 Holcomb Street
Hartford, CT 06112
860-242-2274
https://oakhillct.org/Services-by-Disability/Blind-Visual-Impairments

Lions Clubs International
https://directory.lionsclubs.org/?language=EN

State Office for National Library Services (NLS)
Connecticut State Library
Library for the Blind and Physically Handicapped
198 West Street
Rocky Hill, CT 06067-3554
860-721-2020

http://www.ctstatelibrary.org/organizational-unit/library-blind-physically-handicapped

Delaware

State Agency for the Blind and Visually Impaired

Delaware Department of Health and Social Services: Division for the Visually Impaired
1901 N. Dupont Highway
Biggs Building
New Castle, DE 19720
302-255-9800
http://dhss.delaware.gov/dhss/dvi/

State Office—VA Visual Impairment Services Team (VIST)

Wilmington VAMC
1601 Kirkwood Highway
Wilmington, DE 19805
302-994-2511, x4960

American Optometric Association

http://www.aoa.org/doctor-locator-search?tab=basic&sso=y

American Academy of Ophthalmology

https://secure.aao.org/aao/find-ophthalmologist

NEI's National Eye Health Education Program
https://nei.nih.gov/nehep

State Organizations and Businesses Providing Low-Vision Support, Products, and Services
Wilmington Family Eye Care
801 East Newport Pike
Wilmington, DE 19804
302-999-1286
http://wilmingtonfamilyeyecare.com/

Delaware Low Vision Program
http://www.dhss.delaware.gov/dvi/lowvision.html

Lions Clubs International
https://directory.lionsclubs.org/?language=EN

State Office for National Library Services (NLS)
Delaware Division of Libraries
Delaware Library Access Services
121 Martin Luther King Jr. Boulevard North
Dover, DE 19901-0000
302-739-4748
http://libraries.delaware.gov/dlas.shtml

DISTRICT OF COLUMBIA

State Agency for the Blind and Visually Impaired

District of Columbia Department of Human Services: Rehabilitation Services Administration
1125 Fifteenth Street NW
Washington, DC 20005
202-730-1700
http://dds.dc.gov/service/services-people-blindness-and-visual-impairments

State Office—VA Visual Impairment Services Team (VIST)

Washington DC, VAMC
50 Irving Street NW
Washington, DC 20422
202-745-8000, x55398

American Optometric Association

http://www.aoa.org/doctor-locator-search?tab=basic&sso=y

American Academy of Ophthalmology

https://secure.aao.org/aao/find-ophthalmologist

NEI's National Eye Health Education Program

https://nei.nih.gov/nehep

State Organizations and Businesses Providing Low-Vision Support, Products, and Services

American Foundation for the Blind Public Policy and Research Center
1660 L Street NW, Suite 513
Washington, DC 20036
202-469-6831
http://www.afb.org/info/living-with-vision-loss/1

Columbia Lighthouse for the Blind
1825 K Street NW, Suite 1103
Washington, DC 20006
202-454-6400
http://www.clb.org

Low Vision Center
4905 Del Ray Avenue, Suite 504
Bethesda, MD 20814
301-951-4444
http://www.lowvisioninfo.org/

Lions Clubs International

https://directory.lionsclubs.org/?language=EN

State Office for National Library Services (NLS)

DC Talking Book & Braille Library
Center for Accessibility, DC Public Library

901 G Street NW, Room 215
Washington, DC 20001-0000
202-727-2142
http://dclibrary.org/services/accessibility

Library of Congress National Library Service for the Blind and Physically Handicapped
1291 Taylor Street NW
Washington, DC 20542
202-707-5100
http://www.loc.gov/nls

Florida

State Agency for the Blind and Visually Impaired

Florida Department of Education: Division of Blind Services
325 W. Gaines Street, Suite 1114
Tallahassee, FL 32399
850-245-0331
http://dbs.myflorida.com

State Office—VA Visual Impairment Services Team (VIST)

Bay Pines VA Healthcare System
10000 Bay Pines Boulevard
Bay Pines, FL 33744
727-398-6661, x14516

Lee County Healthcare Center
2489 Diplomat Parkway East
Cape Coral, FL 33909
239-652-1800 x20828

Lee County Healthcare Center
2489 Diplomat Parkway East
Cape Coral, FL 33909
239-652-1800

Miami VA Healthcare System
1201 NW Sixteenth Street
Miami, FL 33125
305-324-4455, x3607

Broward Vo VA OPC
9800 W. Commercial Boulevard
Sunrise, FL 33351
954-625-8730

548 West Palm Beach VAMC
7305 N. Military Trail
West Palm Beach, FL 33410
561-422-8645

Malcom Randall VAMC NF/SGVHS
1601 SW Archer Road

Gainesville, FL 32608
352-376-1611, x5560

Lake City VAMC, NF/SGVHS
619 S. Marion Avenue
Lake City, FL 32025
386-755-3016, x2088

Jacksonville OPC
1536 N. Jefferson Street
Jacksonville, FL 32209
904-475-5868

Tallahassee OPC
1607 St. James Court
Tallahassee, FL 32308
386-755-3016

James A. Haley Veterans' Hospital
10770 North 46th St
Eye Clinic Bldg. (Room F-10)
Tampa, FL 33617
813-903-2442

James A. Haley Veterans' Hospital
10770 North 46th St
Eye Clinic Bldg. (Room F-123)

Tampa, FL 33617
813-903-2414

Orlando VAMC
(11P) Gold Team Rm. 1426
5201 Raymond St
Orlando, FL 32803
407-631-2101

William V. Chappell, Jr.
VA OPC 551
National Health Care Drive
Daytona Beach, FL 32114
386-323-7534

Joint Ambulatory Care Clinic
790 Veterans Way
Pensacola, FL 32507
850-912-2552

American Optometric Association
http://www.aoa.org/doctor-locator-search?tab=basic&sso=y

American Academy of Ophthalmology
https://secure.aao.org/aao/find-ophthalmologist

NEI's National Eye Health Education Program
https://nei.nih.gov/nehep

State Organizations and Businesses Providing Low-Vision Support, Products, and Services
Lighthouse for the Blind of the Palm Beaches
1710 Tiffany Drive East
West Palm Beach, FL 33407
561-586-5600
http://www.lighthousepalmbeaches.org/LowVisionServices

Lighthouse for the Visually Impaired and Blind Inc.
8610 Galen Wilson Boulevard
Port Richey, FL 34668
727-815-0303
http://www.lvib.org/vision-store/

Lighthouse of Broward County
650 N. Andrews Avenue
Ft. Lauderdale, FL 33311
954-463-4217
http://www.lhob.org/low-vision-clinic/services/low-vision-clinic

Florida Reading & Vision Technology Inc. at Lighthouse of Broward

650 N. Andrews Avenue
Fort Lauderdale, Florida 33311
800-981-5119
http://www.floridareading.com/

Lighthouse of Southwest Florida Inc.
35 W. Mariana Avenue
North Fort Myers, FL 33918-5515
239-997-7797
http://lighthouseswfl.org/services/low-vision-program/

Miami Lighthouse for the Blind and Visually Impaired Inc.
601 SW Eighth Avenue
Miami, FL 33130
305-856-2288
http://miamilighthouse.org/LowVisionClinic.asp

Tampa Lighthouse for the Blind
1106 W. Platt Street
Tampa, FL 33606
813-251-2407
http://www.tampalighthouse.org/low-vision-clinic

Lions Clubs International
https://directory.lionsclubs.org/?language=EN

State Office for National Library Services (NLS)

Florida Bureau of Braille and Talking Book Library Services
421 Platt Street
Daytona Beach, FL 32114-2803
386-239-6000
http://dbs.myflorida.com/Talking Books Library/index.html
Serves: Florida - entire state, all 67 counties.

Talking Books/Special Needs Library
Jacksonville Public Library
303 N. Laura Street
Jacksonville, FL 32202-0000
904-630-1999
http://www.jaxpubliclibrary.org/services/talking-books
Serves: Duval County

Talking Books Library
Miami-Dade Public Library System
2455 NW 183rd Street
Miami Gardens, FL 33056-3641
305-751-8687
http://www.mdpls.org/special-services/talking-books.html
Serves: Miami-Dade and Monroe counties

Orange County Library System
Talking Book Section
101 E. Central Boulevard
Orlando, FL 32801-0000
407-835-7464
Serves: Orange County

Talking Books
Palm Beach County Library Annex
4289 Cherry Road
West Palm Beach, FL 33409-9808
561-649-5486
http://www.pbclibrary.org/services/talking-books
Serves: Palm Beach County
Broward County Talking Book Library
100 S. Andrews Avenue
Ft. Lauderdale, FL 33301-1826
954-357-7555
http://www.broward.org/LIBRARY/MYLIBRARYONLINE/Pages/TalkingBookLibrary.aspx
Serves: Broward County

Lee County Talking Books Library
1651 Lee Street
Fort Myers, FL 33901-2916

239-995-2665 or 239-533-4782
https://www.leegov.com/library/about/branches/tb
Serves: Lee County

Brevard County Talking Books Library
Talking Books Library
308 Forrest Avenue
Cocoa, FL 32922-7781
321-633-1810
http://www.brevardcounty.us/publiclibraries
Serves: Brevard County

West Florida Public Library, Talking Books Library
5740 N. Ninth Avenue
Pensacola, FL 32504-0000
850-471-6000 or 850-494-7373
http://www.mywfpl.com
Serves: Escambia County (no longer serving Santa Rosa County)
Pinellas Public Library Cooperative
1330 Cleveland Street
Clearwater, FL 33755-5103
727-441-9958
http://www.pplc.us/tbl/
Serves: Pinellas and Sarasota counties

Georgia

State Agency for the Blind and Visually Impaired

Georgia Department of Labor, Vocational Rehabilitation Program
2 Peachtree Street NW
Atlanta, GA 30303
404-232-1998
http://gvra.georgia.gov/vocationalrehab/

State Office—VA Visual Impairment Services Team (VIST)

Atlanta VAMC
1670 Clairmont Road
Decatur, GA 30033
404-728-4830

Charlie Norwood VAMC
1 Freedom Way
Augusta, GA 30904
706-733-0188, x7573

Carl Vinson VAMC
1826 Veterans Boulevard
Dublin, GA 31021
478-277-2718

American Optometric Association
http://www.aoa.org/doctor-locator-search?tab=basic&sso=y

American Academy of Ophthalmology
https://secure.aao.org/aao/find-ophthalmologist

NEI's National Eye Health Education Program
https://nei.nih.gov/nehep

State Organizations and Businesses Providing Low-Vision Support, Products, and Services
Center for the Visually Impaired
739 W. Peachtree Street NW
Atlanta, GA 30308
404-875-9011
http://www.cviga.org/visability_store/

Medical Center at Augusta University
Eye Clinic
1120 Fifteenth Street
Augusta, GA 30912-5563
706-721-0211
http://www.augustahealth.org/patient-family-centered-care/advisory-councils/eye-clinic

Savannah Center for Blind and Low Vision, previously Savannah Association for the Blind
1141 Cornell Avenue
Savannah, GA 31406
912-236-4473
http://www.savannahcblv.org

Lions Clubs International
https://directory.lionsclubs.org/?language=EN

State Office for National Library Services (NLS)
Georgia Libraries for Accessible Statewide Service
GLASS Distribution Center
5800 Jonesboro Road
Morrow, GA 30260-0000
404-657-1452
http://georgialibraries.org/glass/
Serves: Georgia, except for counties served by subregional libraries; braille readers receive service from Utah.

Southwest Library for Accessible Services
Southwest Georgia Regional Library
301 S. Monroe Street
Bainbridge, GA 39819-4029
229-248-2680
http://www.swgrl.org/handicap.php

Serves: Baker, Brooks, Calhoun, Clay, Colquitt, Decatur, Dougherty, Early, Echols, Grady, Lanier, Lee, Lowndes, Miller, Mitchell, Quitman, Randolph, Seminole, Terrell, Thomas, Webster, and Worth counties

Guam

State Agency for the Blind and Visually Impaired
Guam Department of Integrated Services for Individuals with Disabilities/Division of Vocational Rehabilitation
238 AFC Flores Street, PNB Suite 602
Hagåtña, GU 96910
671-475-4637
http://disid.guam.gov/

State Office—VA Visual Impairment Services Team (VIST)
Guam Vet Center
222 Chalan Santo Papa Street, Suite 201
Hagåtña, GU 96910
671-472-7161

American Optometric Association
http://www.aoa.org/doctor-locator-search?tab=basic&sso=y

American Academy of Ophthalmology
https://secure.aao.org/aao/find-ophthalmologist

NEI's National Eye Health Education Program
https://nei.nih.gov/nehep

State Organizations and Businesses Providing Low-Vision Support, Products, and Services
Seventh Day Adventist Eye Clinic
388 Ypao Road
Tamuning, Guam 96913
671-647-0235
http://www.adventistclinic.com/eye-clinic/

Lions Clubs International
https://directory.lionsclubs.org/?language=EN

State Office for National Library Services (NLS)
Guam Public Library for the Blind and Physically Handicapped
Nieves M. Flores Memorial Library
254 Martyr Street
Agana, GU 96910
671-475-4753
http://gpls.guam.gov/

Hawaii

State Agency for the Blind and Visually Impaired
Hawaii Department of Human Services: Ho'opono Services for the Blind, Division of Vocational Rehabilitation

1901 Bachelot Street
Honolulu, HI 96817
808-586-5269
http://humanservices.hawaii.gov/vr/hoopono/hoopono-services/

State Office—VA Visual Impairment Services Team (VIST)
VA Pacific Islands HCS
459 Patterson Road
Honolulu, HI 96819
808-433-0159

American Optometric Association
http://www.aoa.org/doctor-locator-search?tab=basic&sso=y

American Academy of Ophthalmology
https://secure.aao.org/aao/find-ophthalmologist

NEI's National Eye Health Education Program
https://nei.nih.gov/nehep

State Organizations and Businesses Providing Low-Vision Support, Products, and Services
Hawaii Eye Institute
1380 Lusitana Street, Suite 604
Honolulu, Hawaii 96813

808-523-2020
http://www.hawaii2020.com/low-vision.htm

Hawaiian Eye Center—Wahiawa
606 Kilani Avenue
Wahiawa, HI 96786
808-621-8448

Hawaiian Eye Center—Waipahu
94-307 Farrington Highway, Suite B7-A
Waipahu, HI 96797
808-678-0622
http://www.hawaiianeye.com/eye-conditions/low-vision/

Assistive Technology Resource Centers of Hawaii
200 N. Vineyard Boulevard, Suite 430
Honolulu, HI 96817
808-532-7110
http://www.atrc.org

Lions Clubs International
https://directory.lionsclubs.org/?language=EN

State Office for National Library Services (NLS)
Hawaii Library for the Blind and Physically Handicapped
402 Kapahulu Avenue

Honolulu, HI 96815-3848
808-733-8444
http://www.librarieshawaii.org/lbph

Idaho

State Agency for the Blind and Visually Impaired

Idaho Commission for the Blind
341 W. Washington Street
PO Box 83720
Boise, ID 83720-0012
208-334-3220
http://www.icbvi.state.id.us/

State Office—VA Visual Impairment Services Team (VIST)

Boise VAMC
500 W. Fort Street
Boise, ID 83702
208-422-1228

American Optometric Association

http://www.aoa.org/doctor-locator-search?tab=basic&sso=y

American Academy of Ophthalmology

https://secure.aao.org/aao/find-ophthalmologist

NEI's National Eye Health Education Program
https://nei.nih.gov/nehep

State Organizations and Businesses Providing Low-Vision Support, Products, and Services
Idaho Lions Vision Clinic
1090 N. Cole Road
Boise, ID 83704
208-338-5466
https://www.idaholions.org/vision-clinic-assistance/

Idaho Low Vision Clinic
341 W. Washington St.
Boise, ID 83720-0012
208-334-3220
http://www.icbvi.state.id.us/Low%20Vision%20Clinic.aspx

Lions Clubs International
https://directory.lionsclubs.org/?language=EN

State Office for National Library Services (NLS)
Idaho Commission for Libraries Talking Book Service
325 W. State Street
Boise, ID 83702-6072
208-334-2150
http://libraries.idaho.gov/tbs

ILLINOIS

State Agency for the Blind and Visually Impaired

Illinois Department of Human Services/Division of Rehabilitation Services: Bureau of Blind Services & Business Enterprise Program for the Blind
Bureau of Customer Support and Services
100 S. Grand Avenue East
Springfield, IL 62762
217-785-3887
http://www.dhs.state.il.us/page.aspx?item=32305

State Office—VA Visual Impairment Services Team (VIST)

Jesse Brown VAMC
820 S. Damen Avenue
Chicago, IL 60612
312-569-7531

VA Illiana Health Care System
1900 E. Main Street
Danville, IL 61832
317-554-5406

James A. Lovell FHCC
3001 Green Bay Road
North Chicago, IL 60064
224-610-7168

Edward Hines Jr. VA Hospital
5000 Fifth Avenue
Hines, IL 60141
708-202-2351

Marion VAMC
2401 W. Main Street
Marion, IL 62959
618-997-5311, x54815

American Optometric Association
http://www.aoa.org/doctor-locator-search?tab=basic&sso=y

American Academy of Ophthalmology
https://secure.aao.org/aao/find-ophthalmologist

NEI's National Eye Health Education Program
https://nei.nih.gov/nehep

State Organizations and Businesses Providing Low-Vision Support, Products, and Services
Chicago Lighthouse for People Who Are Blind or Visually Impaired
Vision Care
1850 W. Roosevelt Road
Chicago, IL 60608

312-666-1331
http://chicagolighthouse.org/clinic-locations/

Alfred and Sarah Rosenbloom Center on Vision and Aging
3241 S. Michigan Avenue
Chicago, Illinois 60616
312-949-7250
http://www.illinoiseyeinstitute.org/services/alfred-and-sarah-rosenbloom-center-on-vision-and-aging/

Loyola University Medical Center: Ophthalmology Clinic
2160 S. First Avenue
Maywood, IL 60153
708-216-3833
https://www.loyolamedicine.org/ophthalmology/low-vision-and-vision-rehabilitation

Mary Bryant Home for the Blind
Low Vision Store
2960 Stanton Street
Springfield, IL 62703
217-529-1611
http://www.marybryanthome.org/low-vision-store

Spectrios Institute for Low Vision
(formerly Deicke Center for Visual Rehabilitation)

219 E. Cole Avenue
Wheaton, IL 60187
630-690-7115
http://www.spectrios.org

TCRC Sight Center
81A E. Queenwood Road
Morton, IL 61550
309-291-0573
http://www.tcrcorg.com/facilities/

Lions Clubs International
https://directory.lionsclubs.org/?language=EN

State Office for National Library Services (NLS)
Illinois State Library Talking Book and Braille Service
300 S. Second Street
Springfield, IL 62701-1796
217-782-9435
http://www.ilbph.org
Serves: Illinois

Illinois Taking Book Outreach Center
Reaching Across Illinois Library System
125 Tower Drive
Burr Ridge, IL 60527-5783

630-734-5210
http://www.illinoistalkingbooks.org

INDIANA

State Agency for the Blind and Visually Impaired

Indiana Family and Social Services Administration: Division of Disability and Rehabilitative Services, Blind and Visually Impaired Services
Indiana Government Center
402 W. Washington Street, Room W453
Indianapolis, IN 46207
317-232-1441
http://www.in.gov/fssa/ddrs/2638.htm

State Office—VA Visual Impairment Services Team (VIST)

Richard L. Roudebush VAMC (Indianapolis VAMC)
1481 W. Tenth Street
Indianapolis, IN 46202
317-988-2566

VA Northern Indiana HCS
Fort Wayne Campus
2121 Lake Avenue
Fort Wayne, IN 46805
260-426-5431, x72650

American Optometric Association
http://www.aoa.org/doctor-locator-search?tab=basic&sso=y

American Academy of Ophthalmology
https://secure.aao.org/aao/find-ophthalmologist

NEI's National Eye Health Education Program
https://nei.nih.gov/nehep

State Organizations and Businesses Providing Low-Vision Support, Products, and Services
Evansville Association for the Blind
500 N. Second Avenue
Evansville, IN 47710
812-422-1181
http://www.evansvilleblind.org/how-we-serve/low-vision/

Indiana University School of Optometry: Eye Care Centers
Atwater Eye Care Center (Bloomington, Indiana)
812-855-8436
Indianapolis Eye Care Center (Indianapolis, Indiana)
317-321-1470
http://www.optometry.iu.edu/clinics/locations/index.shtml

League for the Blind and Disabled Inc.
5821 S. Anthony Boulevard
Fort Wayne, IN 46816

260-441-0551
https://www.the-league.org/services/senior-blind-services-55/

Lions Clubs International
https://directory.lionsclubs.org/?language=EN

State Office for National Library Services (NLS)
Indiana State Library
Indiana Talking Book & Braille Library
140 N. Senate Avenue
Indianapolis, IN 46204-0000
317-232-3684
http://www.in.gov/library/tbbl.htm
Serves: Indiana

Bartholomew County Public Library
Talking Book Service
536 Fifth Street
Columbus, IN 47201-0000
812-379-1277
http://www.barth.lib.in.us/talkingbooks.html
Serves: Bartholomew, Clark, Crawford, Decatur, Floyd, Harrison, Jackson, Jefferson, Jennings, Scott, and Washington counties

Northwest Indiana Subregional Library for the Blind and Physically Handicapped

Lake County Public Library
1919 W. Eighty-First Avenue
Merrillville, IN 46410-5382
219-769-3541
http://www.lcplin.org/read/talking-books.html
Serves: Jasper, Lake, LaPorte, Newton, and Porter counties

Talking Books Service
Evansville-Vanderburgh Public Library
200 SE Martin Luther King Jr. Boulevard
Evansville, IN 47713-1802
812-428-8235
http://evpl.org/services/tbs/
Serves: Daviess, Dubois, Gibson, Knox, Martin, Perry, Pike, Posey, Spencer, Vanderburgh, and Warrick counties

Iowa

State Agency for the Blind and Visually Impaired

Iowa Department for the Blind
524 Fourth Street
Des Moines, IA 50309-2364
515-281-1333
https://blind.iowa.gov/

State Office—VA Visual Impairment Services Team (VIST)

Des Moines Division—VA Central Iowa Health Care System
3600 Thirtieth Street
Des Moines, IA 50310
515-699-5410

Iowa City VAMC
601 Highway 6 West
Iowa City, IA 52246
319 338-0581, x6889

American Optometric Association

http://www.aoa.org/doctor-locator-search?tab=basic&sso=y

American Academy of Ophthalmology

https://secure.aao.org/aao/find-ophthalmologist

NEI's National Eye Health Education Program

https://nei.nih.gov/nehep

State Organizations and Businesses Providing Low-Vision Support, Products, and Services

University of Iowa Hospitals and Clinics: Vision Rehabilitation Service
200 Hawkins Drive, 11190A PFP
University of Iowa Carver College of Medicine

Department of Ophthalmology and Visual Sciences
Iowa City, IA 52242
319-356-8301
https://www.medicine.uiowa.edu/eye/

NanoPac Inc.
4823 S. Sheridan Road, Suite 302
Tulsa, OK 74145
800-580-6086
http://www.nanopac.com/

Wolfe Eye Clinic
Ames, Cedar Falls, Cedar Rapids, Des Moines, Fort Dodge, Iowa City, Marshalltown, Ottumwa, Spencer, and Waterloo
800-542-7956
http://www.wolfeeyeclinic.com/locations

Broadlawns Eye Clinic
1801 Hickman Road
Des Moines, IA 50314-1597
515-282-2200
http://www.broadlawns.org/eye-clinic.cfm

Vision Specialists of Council Bluffs
1505 West Broadway Suite 3-5
Council Bluffs, IA 51501

712-322-3097
http://visionsource-vsofcb.com/

Des Moines Eye Surgeons
5901 Westown Parkway Suite 200
West Des Moines, IA 50266
515-225-3546
http://www.dmeyesurgeons.com/

Family Eyecare Centers
1601 Avenue 'D'
Council Bluffs, IA 51501
712-323-5213
http://www.familyeyecare.biz/

Mauer Eye Center
2515 Cyclone Drive
Waterloo, Iowa 50701
319-433-3000
http://mauereye.com/

Ankeny Family Vision Center
311 N. Ankeny Boulevard
Ankeny, IA 50023
515-964-1671
http://www.afvcweb.com/

Iowa Radio Reading Information Service
for the Blind and Print Handicapped, Inc.
100 East Euclid Avenue, Suite 117
Des Moines, Iowa 50313
515-243-6833
http://www.iowaradioreading.org/

Tri-State Independent Blind Society Inc.
3333 Asbury Road
Dubuque, Iowa 52001
563-556-8746
http://www.tristateblind.org/low.php

Iowa Low Vision
PO Box 1533
Council Bluffs, IA 51502
515-218-8024
http://www.IowaLowVision.com/

Lions Clubs International
https://directory.lionsclubs.org/?language=EN

State Office for National Library Services (NLS)
Iowa Library for the Blind and Physically Handicapped
Iowa Department for the Blind
524 Fourth Street
Des Moines, IA 50309-2364

515-281-1368
https://blind.iowa.gov/library
Serves: Iowa

KANSAS

State Agency for the Blind and Visually Impaired

Kansas Department for Children and Families: Services for People Who Are Blind or Visually Impaired
555 S. Third Floor
Topeka, KS 66603
785-368-7471
http://www.dcf.ks.gov/services/RS/Pages/Blind.aspx

State Office—VA Visual Impairment Services Team (VIST)

VA Eastern Kansas Health Care System—Dwight D. Eisenhower VAMC
4101 S. Fourth Street
Leavenworth, KS 66048
913-682-2000, x52657

Robert J. Dole Medical and Regional Office Center
5500 E. Kellogg Avenue
Wichita, KS 67218
316-651-3682

American Optometric Association
http://www.aoa.org/doctor-locator-search?tab=basic&sso=y

American Academy of Ophthalmology
https://secure.aao.org/aao/find-ophthalmologist

NEI's National Eye Health Education Program
https://nei.nih.gov/nehep

State Organizations and Businesses Providing Low-Vision Support, Products, and Services
NanoPac Inc.
4823 S. Sheridan Road, Suite 302
Tulsa, OK 74145
800-580-6086
http://www.nanopac.com/

Bicknell Envision Vision Rehabilitation Center
610 N. Main Street
Wichita, KS 67203
316-440-1600
http://www.envisionus.com/How-We-Help/Rehabilitation-Therapy

Kansas City Eye Clinic
7504 Antioch Road
Overland Park, KS 66204

913-341-3100
https://www.kceyeclinic.com/our-services/low-vision/

Lifetime Eyecare
105 South Penn Ave
Oberlin, KS 67749
785-475-1200
http://lecvisionsource.com/

Fry Eye Associates
Western Kansas Low Vision
310 E. Walnut Street
Garden City, KS 67846
620-275-7248
http://www.fryeye.com/lowvision.htm

Lions Clubs International
https://directory.lionsclubs.org/?language=EN

State Office for National Library Services (NLS)
Kansas State Library
Kansas Talking Books Regional Library—Box 4055
ESU
1 Kellogg Circle
Emporia, KS 66801-5415
620-341-6280

http://www.kslib.info/talking
Serves: Kansas; braille readers receive service from Utah.

NW Kansas Library System
Advisory and Outreach Center
2 Washington Square
Norton, KS 67654-0000
785-877-5148
http://nwkls.org/western-kansas-talking-books/
Serves: Cheyenne, Decatur, Gove, Graham, Logan, Norton, Rawlins, Sheridan, Sherman, Thomas, and Trego counties

Central Kansas Library System
Advisory and Outreach Center
1409 Williams Street
Great Bend, KS 67530-0000
620-792-2393
http://ckls.org/services/talking-books/
Serves: Barton, Cloud, Ellis, Ellsworth, Jewel, Lincoln, Mitchel, Osborne, Ottawa, Pawnee, Phillips, Republic, Rooks, Rush, Russell, Salina, and Smith counties

Kentucky

State Agency for the Blind and Visually Impaired

Kentucky Office for the Blind

275 E. Main Street
Mail Stop 2-EJ
Frankfort, KY 40621
502-782-3414
http://blind.ky.gov

State Office—VA Visual Impairment Services Team (VIST)
Lexington VAMC
1101 Veterans Drive
Lexington, KY 40502
859-281-3916

Louisville VAMC
800 Zorn Avenue
Louisville, KY 40206
502-287-4000, x55049

American Optometric Association
http://www.aoa.org/doctor-locator-search?tab=basic&sso=y

American Academy of Ophthalmology
https://secure.aao.org/aao/find-ophthalmologist

NEI's National Eye Health Education Program
https://nei.nih.gov/nehep

State Organizations and Businesses Providing Low-Vision Support, Products, and Services

Retina Associates of Kentucky
120 N. Eagle Creek Drive, Suite 500
Lexington, KY 40509
859-263-3900
Louisville Office
6420 Dutchman's Lane, Suite 70
Louisville, KY 40205
502-895-2600
http://www.retinaky.com/Low_Vision_Services/

Kentucky Lions Eye Center: Low Vision Clinic
University of Louisville Department of Ophthalmology
301 E. Muhammad Ali Boulevard
Louisville, KY 40202
502-583-0550
https://www.uoflphysicians.com/ky-lions-eye-center

Lions Clubs International

https://directory.lionsclubs.org/?language=EN

State Office for National Library Services (NLS)

Kentucky Talking Book Library
300 Coffee Tree Road
PO Box 537
Frankfort, KY 40602-0537

502-564-5791
http://kdla.ky.gov/librarians/talkingbook
Serves: Kentucky

LOUISIANA

State Agency for the Blind and Visually Impaired

Louisiana Department of Social Services: Rehabilitation Services
627 N. Fourth Street
Baton Rouge, LA 70802
225-219-2943
http://www.dss.state.la.us/

State Office—VA Visual Impairment Services Team (VIST)

Alexandria VAMC
PO Box 69004
Alexandria, LA 71306
318-473-0010, x2047

Southeast Louisiana Veterans Health Care System
1601 Perdido Street
New Orleans, LA 70112
504-506-8400, x7215

Overton Brooks VAMC
510 E. Stoner Avenue

Shreveport, LA 71101
318-990-4839

American Optometric Association
http://www.aoa.org/doctor-locator-search?tab=basic&sso=y

American Academy of Ophthalmology
https://secure.aao.org/aao/find-ophthalmologist

NEI's National Eye Health Education Program
https://nei.nih.gov/nehep

State Organizations and Businesses Providing Low-Vision Support, Products, and Services
Louisiana Rehabilitation Services
950 N. Twenty-Second Street
Baton Rouge, LA 70802
225-219-2943
http://www.laworks.net/WorkforceDev/LRS/LRS_BlindServices.asp

Lighthouse for the Blind in New Orleans
123 State Street
New Orleans, LA 70118
504-899-4501
http://lighthouse-louisiana.myshopify.com/collections/magnifiers-more

Louisiana Association for the Blind
Low Vision Rehabilitation Center
1750 Claiborne Avenue
Shreveport, LA 71103
318-635-6471
https://lablind.com/lowvision.php

Lions Clubs International
https://directory.lionsclubs.org/?language=EN

State Office for National Library Services (NLS)
State Library of Louisiana
Talking Books and Braille Library
701 N. Fourth Street
Baton Rouge, LA 70802-5232
225-342-0035
http://www.state.lib.la.us/special-services/tbbl
Serves: Louisiana; braille readers receive service from Utah.

Maine

State Agency for the Blind and Visually Impaired
Maine Department of Labor: Division for the Blind and Visually Impaired
150 State House Station

Augusta, ME 04333
207-623-6799
http://www.maine.gov/rehab/dbvi/

State Office—VA Visual Impairment Services Team (VIST)
Togus VAMC
1 VA Center
Augusta, ME 04330
207-623-8411, x5944

American Optometric Association
http://www.aoa.org/doctor-locator-search?tab=basic&sso=y

American Academy of Ophthalmology
https://secure.aao.org/aao/find-ophthalmologist

NEI's National Eye Health Education Program
https://nei.nih.gov/nehep

State Organizations and Businesses Providing Low-Vision Support, Products, and Services
Eye Care of Maine
325A Kennedy Memorial Drive
Waterville ME 04901
800-660-3403
http://maine2020.com/low-vision-services/

The Iris Network
189 Park Avenue
Portland, ME 04102
207-774-6273
http://www.theiris.org

Lions Clubs International
https://directory.lionsclubs.org/?language=EN

State Office for National Library Services (NLS)
Library Services for the Blind and Physically Handicapped
Maine State Library
64 State House Station
Augusta, ME 04333-0064
207-287-5650
http://www.maine.gov/msl/outreach/lbph/
Serves: Maine; braille readers receive service from Massachusetts.

Maryland

State Agency for the Blind and Visually Impaired
Maryland State Department of Education: Division of Rehabilitation Services
2301 Argonne Drive
Baltimore, MD 21218-1696

410-554-9277
http://www.dors.maryland.gov

State Office—VA Visual Impairment Services Team (VIST)
Baltimore VAMC—VA Maryland Health Care System
10 N. Greene Street
Baltimore, MD 21201
410-605-7000, x5124

(Lochraven Campus)
LRC-Room 1A-119
Baltimore, MD 21201
410-605-7650 x4498

American Optometric Association
http://www.aoa.org/doctor-locator-search?tab=basic&sso=y

American Academy of Ophthalmology
https://secure.aao.org/aao/find-ophthalmologist

NEI's National Eye Health Education Program
https://nei.nih.gov/nehep

State Organizations and Businesses Providing Low-Vision Support, Products, and Services
Low Vision Center

4905 Del Ray Avenue, Suite 504
Bethesda, MD 20814
301-951-4444
http://www.lowvisioninfo.org

National Federation of the Blind
200 E. Wells Street at Jernigan Place
Baltimore, MD 21230
410-659-9314
https://nfb.org/information-about-vision-loss

National Institutes of Health: National Eye Institute
31 Center Drive
MSC 2510
Bethesda, MD 20892-2510
301-496-5248
http://www.nei.nih.gov

Walter Reed Army Medical Center: Ophthalmology Service
8901 Rockville Pike
Building 8, Floor 1
Bethesda, MD 20889
301-295-1339
http://www.wrnmmc.capmed.mil/Health%20Services/Surgery/Surgery/Ophthalmology/SitePages/Home.aspx

Wilmer Eye Institute
Johns Hopkins Hospital
600 N. Wolfe Street
Baltimore, MD 21287
410-955-0580
http://www.wilmereyeinstitute.org

American Macular Degeneration Foundation
PO Box 515
Northampton, MA 01061-0515
413-268-7660
http://www.macular.org/

Boston University Eye Associates
2005 Bay Street, Suite 201
Taunton, MA 02780
508-823-7473
http://buea.net/

Carroll Center for the Blind
770 Centre Street
Newton, MA 02458-2597
617-969-6200
http://carroll.org/services/vision-assessments/

Lions Clubs International
https://directory.lionsclubs.org/?language=EN

State Office for National Library Services (NLS)
Maryland State Library for the Blind and Physically Handicapped
415 Park Avenue
Baltimore, MD 21201-3603
410-230-2424
http://www.lbph.lib.md.us
Serves: Maryland

MASSACHUSETTS

State Agency for the Blind and Visually Impaired
Massachusetts Commission for the Blind
600 Washington Street
Boston, MA 02111
617-727-5550
http://www.mass.gov/mcb

State Office—VA Visual Impairment Services Team (VIST)
Edith Nourse Rogers Memorial Veterans Hospital
200 Springs Road
Bedford, MA 01730
781-687-2705

VA Boston HCS, Jamaica Plain Campus
150 S. Huntington Avenue

Jamaica Plain, MA 02130
857-364-6555
857-364-2283

VA Central Western Massachusetts Healthcare System
421 N. Main Street
Leeds, MA 01053
413-584-4040, x2058

American Optometric Association
http://www.aoa.org/doctor-locator-search?tab=basic&sso=y

American Academy of Ophthalmology
https://secure.aao.org/aao/find-ophthalmologist

NEI's National Eye Health Education Program
https://nei.nih.gov/nehep

State Organizations and Businesses Providing Low-Vision Support, Products, and Services
Massachusetts Eye and Ear Infirmary: Vision Rehabilitation Center
243 Charles Street, Eighth Floor
Boston, MA 02114
617-573-4177
http://www.meei.harvard.edu/specialties/ophthalmology/vision-rehabilitation-service

New England Eye Commonwealth
930 Commonwealth Avenue West, Suite 2A
Boston, MA 02215
617-262-2020
http://www.neco.edu/patient-care/about-nee

New England Eye Roslindale
Roslindale Square
4199 Washington Street, Suite 2
Roslindale, MA 02131
617-323-7300
http://www.newenglandeye.org/our-locations/roslindale

New England Eye Southeastern Massachusetts (SEMA)
450 Pleasant Street
East Bridgewater, MA 02333
617-680-8447
http://www.newenglandeye.org/our-locations/sema

New England Eye Low Vision Clinic at Perkins
Perkins School for the Blind
175 N. Beacon Street
Watertown, MA 02472
617-972-7296
http://www.perkins.org/school/public/low-vision-clinic?gclid=CLiW8OW9ydACFcolgQodqwgliA

Lions Clubs International
https://directory.lionsclubs.org/?language=EN

State Office for National Library Services (NLS)
Perkins Library
Perkins School for the Blind
175 N. Beacon Street
Watertown, MA 02472-2790
617-972-7240
http://www.perkinslibrary.org
Serves: Massachusetts

Worcester Talking Book Library
Worcester Public Library
3 Salem Square
Worcester, MA 01608-2074
508-799-1730
http://talkingbook.mywpl.org
Serves: Worcester Talking Book Library serves Massachusetts.

Michigan

State Agency for the Blind and Visually Impaired
Bureau of Services for Blind Persons, Michigan Department of Licensing and Regulatory Affairs
201 N. Washington Square
Lansing, MI 48933

517-373-2062
www.michigan.gov/BSBP

State Office—VA Visual Impairment Services Team (VIST)
VA Ann Arbor Healthcare System
2215 Fuller Road
Ann Arbor, MI 48105
734-845-3064

Battle Creek VAMC
5500 Armstrong Road
Battle Creek, MI 49015
269-223-6607

John D. Dingell VAMC
4646 John R Street
Detroit, MI 48201
313-576-1000, x64888

Aleda E. Lutz VAMC
1500 Weiss Street
Saginaw, MI 48602
989-497-2500, x11852

Iron Mountain VAMC
325 E. H Street

Iron Mountain, MI 49801
906-774-3300, x34515

American Optometric Association
http://www.aoa.org/doctor-locator-search?tab=basic&sso=y

American Academy of Ophthalmology
https://secure.aao.org/aao/find-ophthalmologist

NEI's National Eye Health Education Program
https://nei.nih.gov/nehep

State Organizations and Businesses Providing Low-Vision Support, Products, and Services
Association for the Blind and Visually Impaired
456 Cherry Street SE
Grand Rapids, MI 49503
616-458-1187
http://www.abvimichigan.org/what-we-do/low-vision-clinics/

Beaumont Eye Institute: Low Vision Center
3535 W. 13 Mile Road, Suite 555
Royal Oak, MI 48073
248-551-2020
http://www.beaumont.edu/centers-services/rehabilitation-services-and-programs/adult-rehabilitation/neurological/low-vision/

Detroit Institute of Ophthalmology, A division of the Henry Ford Department of Ophthalmology
15415 E. Jefferson Avenue
Grosse Pointe Park, MI 48230
313-824-4710
http://www.henryford.com/DIO

Ferris State University: Michigan College of Optometry, Low Vision Services
1124 S. State Street, MCO 101A
Big Rapids, MI 49307
231-591-2020
http://www.ferris.edu/HTMLS/colleges/michopt/eye-vision-information/low-vision/

Greater Detroit Agency for the Blind and Visually Impaired
16625 Grand River Avenue
Detroit, MI 48227
313-272-3900
http://www.gdabvi.org

Low Vision and Visual Rehabilitative Services: University of Michigan Kellogg Eye Center
University of Michigan Kellogg Eye Center
1000 Wall Street
Ann Arbor, MI 48105

734-764-5106
http://www.kellogg.umich.edu

Western Michigan University: Vision Clinic
Unified Clinics
1000 Oakland Drive, Fourth Floor
Kalamazoo, MI 49008
269-387-7064
http://www.wmich.edu/unifiedclinics/about/vision

Lions Clubs International
https://directory.lionsclubs.org/?language=EN

State Office for National Library Services (NLS)
Michigan Braille and Talking Book Library
702 W. Kalamazoo Street
Lansing, MI 48909
517-373-5614
http://www.michigan.gov/btbl
Serves: Michigan

Washtenaw Library for the Blind & Physically Disabled
@ Ann Arbor District Library
343 S. Fifth Avenue
Ann Arbor, MI 48104-0000
734-327-4200

http://wlbpd.aadl.org
Serves: Washtenaw County

Great Lakes Talking Books Reader Advisory and Outreach Center
1615 Presque Isle Avenue
Marquette, MI 49855-0000
906-228-7697
http://GreatLakesTalkingBooks.org
Serves: Fifteen counties in the Upper Peninsula, Alpena County, and Crawford County

Oakland Talking Book Service @ RHPL
500 Olde Towne Road
Rochester Hills, MI 48307-2043
248-650-5681 or 248-650-7150
http://otbs.rhpl.org
Serves: Oakland County

Genesee District Talking Book Advisory and Outreach Center
Library for the Blind and Physically Handicapped
4195 W. Pasadena Avenue
Flint, MI 48504-2344
810-732-1120
https://www.thegdl.org/services/talking-book-center
Serves: Genesee county

Kent District Advisory and Outreach Center for the Blind and Physically Handicapped
Wyoming Branch Library
3350 Michael Avenue SW
Wyoming, MI 49509-0000
616-647-3988 or 616-784-2016, ext. 4985
http://www.kdl.org/services/lbph
Serves: Ionia, Kent, and Montcalm counties

Traverse Area District Library Advisory and Outreach Center
610 Woodmere Avenue
Traverse City, MI 49686-3397
231-932-8558
http://www.tadl.org/tbl
Serves: Antrim, Benzie, Grand Traverse, Kalkaska, Leelanau, Manistee, Missaukee, and Wexford counties

St. Clair County Library
St. Clair County Library for the Blind and Physically Handicapped
210 McMorran Boulevard
Port Huron, MI 48060-0000
810-982-3600
http://www.sccl.lib.mi.us/LBPH.aspx
Serves: Huron, Sanilac, St. Clair, and Tuscola Counties

Muskegon Area District Library for the Blind and Physically Handicapped
4845 Airline Road, Suite 5
Muskegon, MI 49444-4563
231-737-6310
http://www.madl.org
Serves: Muskegon and Ottawa counties

Macomb Library for the Blind and Physically Handicapped @ CMPL
40900 Romeo Plank Road
Clinton Township, MI 48038-2955
586-286-1580
http://www.cmpl.org/mlbph/
Serves: Macomb County

Braille and Talking Books @ Taylor Community Library
12303 Pardee Road
Taylor, MI 48180
734-287-4840
http://www.taylor.lib.mi.us
Serves: Wayne County except Detroit
Detroit Library for the Blind and Physically Handicapped
Detroit Public Library
Frederick Douglass Branch for Specialized Services
3666 Grand River Avenue
Detroit, MI 48208-0000

313-481-1702
http://www.detroitpubliclibrary.org/lbph/LBPH_index.htm
Serves: Detroit and Highland Park (Wayne County)

Minnesota

State Agency for the Blind and Visually Impaired
Minnesota State Services for the Blind
2200 University Avenue West, Suite 240
St. Paul, MN 55114-1840
651-539-2300
http://www.mnssb.org/

State Office—VA Visual Impairment Services Team (VIST)
Minneapolis VAMC
One Veterans Drive
Minneapolis, MN 55417
612-467-2000, x7575

St. Cloud VAMC
4801 Veterans Drive
St. Cloud, MN 56303
320-255-6480, x6192

American Optometric Association
http://www.aoa.org/doctor-locator-search?tab=basic&sso=y

American Academy of Ophthalmology
https://secure.aao.org/aao/find-ophthalmologist

NEI's National Eye Health Education Program
https://nei.nih.gov/nehep

State Organizations and Businesses Providing Low-Vision Support, Products, and Services
Lighthouse Center for Vision Loss
4505 W. Superior Street
Duluth, MN 55807-2728
218-624-4828
http://www.lcfvl.org

Mayo Clinic Department of Ophthalmology: Low Vision Service
Mayo West 7A
200 First Street SW
Rochester, MN 55905
507-284-3726
http://www.mayoclinic.org/ophthalmology-rst/lowvision.html

Regions Hospital: Low Vision Clinic
640 Jackson Street
St. Paul, MN 55101

651-221-3456
http://www.regionshospital.com/

University of Minnesota: Vision Rehabilitation Center
516 Delaware Street SE
Minneapolis, MN 55455-0501
612-625-4400
http://www.ophthalmology.umn.edu/patient-care/find-clinic

Vision Loss Resources—Minneapolis and West Metro
1936 Lyndale Avenue South
Minneapolis, MN 55403
612-871-2222
http://visionlossresources.org/programs/rehabilitation-center

Vision Loss Resources—St. Paul and East Metro
216 S. Wabasha Street
St. Paul, MN 55107
651-224-7662
http://visionlossresources.org/programs/rehabilitation-center

Lions Clubs International
https://directory.lionsclubs.org/?language=EN

State Office for National Library Services (NLS)
Minnesota Braille and Talking Book Library
388 SE Sixth Avenue
Faribault, MN 55021-6340
507-333-4828
http://www.mnbtbl.org
Serves: Minnesota

MISSISSIPPI

State Agency for the Blind and Visually Impaired
Mississippi Department of Rehabilitation Services: Office of Vocational Rehabilitation for the Blind
1281 Highway 51 North
Madison, MS 39110
601-853-5300
http://www.mdrs.ms.gov/VocationalRehabBlind/Pages/default.aspx

State Office—VA Visual Impairment Services Team (VIST)
VA Gulf Coast Veterans Health Care System
400 Veterans Avenue
Biloxi, MS 39531
228-385-6762

G.V. (Sonny) Montgomery VAMC
1500 E. Woodrow Wilson Drive
Jackson, MS 39216
601-362-4471, x5078
601-362-4471, x1551

American Optometric Association
http://www.aoa.org/doctor-locator-search?tab=basic&sso=y

American Academy of Ophthalmology
https://secure.aao.org/aao/find-ophthalmologist

NEI's National Eye Health Education Program
https://nei.nih.gov/nehep

State Organizations and Businesses Providing Low-Vision Support, Products, and Services
Addie McBryde Rehabilitation Center for the Blind
2550 Peachtree Street
Jackson, MS 39296-5314
601-364-2700
http://www.mdrs.ms.gov/VocationalRehabBlind/Pages/Addie_McBryde.aspx

Mississippi State University, The National Research and Training Center on Blindness and Low Vision

PO Box 6189
Mississippi State, MS 39762
662-325-2001
nrtc@colled.msstate.edu
http://www.blind.msstate.edu

Mississippi Industries for the Blind
Low Vision Store
2501 North West Street
Jackson, MS 39216
601-984-3200
http://www.msblind.org/store.htm

University of Mississippi Medical Center: Department of Ophthalmology
2500 N. State Street
Jackson, MS 39216-4505
601-984-5020
https://www.umc.edu/eye/

Lions Clubs International
https://directory.lionsclubs.org/?language=EN

State Office for National Library Services (NLS)
Talking Book Services
Mississippi Library Commission
3881 Eastwood Drive

Jackson, MS 39211-6473
601-432-4111
http://mlc.lib.ms.us/tbs/
Serves: Mississippi; braille readers receive service from Utah

Missouri

State Agency for the Blind and Visually Impaired

Missouri Rehabilitation Services for the Blind
615 Howerton Court
Jefferson City, MO 65102
573-751-4249
http://www.dss.mo.gov/fsd/rsb/

State Office—VA Visual Impairment Services Team (VIST)

Kansas City VAMC
4801 Linwood Boulevard
Kansas City, MO 64128
816-861-4700, x56294

St. Louis VAMC—John Cochran Division
915 N. Grand Boulevard
St. Louis, MO 63106
314-652-4100, x54121

Harry S. Truman Memorial
800 Hospital Drive
Columbia, MO 65201
573-814-6458

Poplar-Bluff VAMC
1500 N. Westwood Boulevard
Poplar Bluff, MO 63901
573-686-4151, x52151

American Optometric Association
http://www.aoa.org/doctor-locator-search?tab=basic&sso=y

American Academy of Ophthalmology
https://secure.aao.org/aao/find-ophthalmologist

NEI's National Eye Health Education Program
https://nei.nih.gov/nehep

State Organizations and Businesses Providing Low-Vision Support, Products, and Services
NanoPac Inc.
4823 S. Sheridan Road, Suite 302
Tulsa, OK 74145
800-580-6086
http://www.nanopac.com/

Alphapointe Low Vision Clinic
7501 Prospect Avenue
Kansas City, MO 64132
816-421-5848
https://www.alphapointe.org/Low%20Vision%20Clinic

Lighthouse for the Blind—St. Louis
10440 Trenton Avenue
St. Louis, MO 63132-1223
314-423-4333
http://www.lhbindustries.com/Our-Outreach/Programs.aspx

St. Louis Society for the Blind and Visually Impaired
8770 Manchester Road
St. Louis, MO 63144
314-968-9000
http://www.slsbvi.org/drews-low-vision-clinic/

Missouri Assistive Technology
1501 NW Jefferson St.
Blue Springs, MO 64015
816-655-6700
http://at.mo.gov/

Mason Eye Institute, Department of Ophthalmology, University of Missouri

University of Missouri
Department of Ophthalmology
One Hospital Drive
Columbia, MO 65212
573-882-1029 (Local)
http://medicine.missouri.edu/ophthalmology/

St. Louis University: Eye Institute
1755 South Grand
St. Louis, MO 63104
314-256-3220
http://medschool.slu.edu/departments/eye/

American Optometric Association: Low Vision Rehabilitation Section
243 North Lindbergh Boulevard
St. Louis, MO 63141
314-991-4100
http://www.aoa.org/patients-and-public/caring-for-your-vision/low-vision/low-vision-rehabilitation?sso=y

Lions Clubs International
https://directory.lionsclubs.org/?language=EN

State Office for National Library Services (NLS)
Wolfner Talking Book and Braille Library

PO Box 387
Jefferson City, MO 65102-0387
573-751-8720
http://www.sos.mo.gov/wolfner
Serves: Missouri

MONTANA

State Agency for the Blind and Visually Impaired

Montana Vocational Rehabilitation and Blind Services
111 N. Last Chance Gulch, Suite 4C
PO Box 4210
Helena, MT 59604
406-444-2590
http://dphhs.mt.gov/detd/blvs/blvs-vr

State Office—VA Visual Impairment Services Team (VIST)

VA Montana Health Care System
1766 Majestic Lane
Billings, MT 59102
406-373-3943

VA Montana Health Care System
3687 Veterans Drive
Fort Harrison, MT 59636
406-874-5843

American Optometric Association
http://www.aoa.org/doctor-locator-search?tab=basic&sso=y

American Academy of Ophthalmology
https://secure.aao.org/aao/find-ophthalmologist

NEI's National Eye Health Education Program
https://nei.nih.gov/nehep

State Organizations and Businesses Providing Low-Vision Support, Products, and Services
Low Vision Montana
PO Box 664
Helena, MT 59624
800-601-5004
http://www.lowvisionmt.org/

Lions Clubs International
https://directory.lionsclubs.org/?language=EN

State Office for National Library Services (NLS)
Montana Talking Book Library
1515 E. Sixth Avenue
PO Box 201800
Helena, MT 59620-1800
406-444-2064 or 406-444-5399

http://tbl.msl.mt.gov
Serves: Montana

NEBRASKA

State Agency for the Blind and Visually Impaired
Nebraska Commission for the Blind and Visually Impaired
4600 Valley Road, Suite 100
Lincoln, NE 68510-4844
402-471-2891
http://www.ncbvi.ne.gov

State Office—VA Visual Impairment Services Team (VIST)
Omaha Division—VA Nebraska Western Iowa Health Care System
4101 Woolworth Avenue
Omaha, NE 68105
402-346-8800, x3188

American Optometric Association
http://www.aoa.org/doctor-locator-search?tab=basic&sso=y

American Academy of Ophthalmology
https://secure.aao.org/aao/find-ophthalmologist

NEI's National Eye Health Education Program
https://nei.nih.gov/nehep

State Organizations and Businesses Providing Low-Vision Support, Products, and Services
The Weigel Williamson Center for Visual Rehabilitation
704 S. Thirty-Eighth Avenue
Omaha, NE 68105
402-559-2463
http://www.unmc.edu/lowvision

Outlook Nebraska Inc.
4125 S. Seventy-Second Street,
Omaha, NE 68127
402-614-3331
https://outlooknebraska.org/

NanoPac Inc.
4823 S. Sheridan Road, Suite 302
Tulsa, OK 74145
800-580-6086
http://www.nanopac.com/

ilumin
16820 Frances Street, Suite 100
Omaha, NE 68130

402-933-6600
http://www.ilumineyes.com/

ilumin
450 Regency Parkway, Suite 110
Omaha, NE 68114
402-933-6600

Eye Consultants, PC Eyeoptics
8141 W. Center Road, Suite 100
Omaha, NE 68124
402-391-1100
http://www.eyeconsultantspc.com/

Heartland Eye Consultants
9900 Nicholas Street, Suite 250
Omaha, NE 68114
402-493-6500
https://heartland-eye.com/

Midwest Eye Care
4353 Dodge Street
Omaha, NE 68131
402-552-2020
http://www.midwesteyecare.com/

Madonna's Low Vision Services
5401 South Street
Lincoln, NE 68506
800-676-5448
https://www.madonna.org/programs-and-services/vision

Nebraska Assistive Technology Partnership
3901 N. Twenty-Seventh Street, Suite 5
Lincoln, NE 68521
402-471-0734
http://www.atp.ne.gov/

Oculi Eye Care and Vision Rehabilitation
1401 Infinity Road, Suite D
Lincoln, Nebraska 68512
402-420-0880
http://oculivision.com/

Advanced Eye Care
1414 W 12th Street
Hastings, NE 68901
402-462-9191
http://www.eyecarehastings.com/

Professional Eye Care
1511 M Street

Ord, NE 68862
308-728-3229
http://visionsource-professionaleyecare.com/

Eye Physicians P.C.
3772 - 43rd Avenue
Columbus, Nebraska 68601
402-563-3686
http://www.eyephysicianspc.com/

Lifetime Eyecare
218 West D Street
McCook, Nebraska 69001
308-345-5800
http://lecvisionsource.com/

Nebraska Low Vision
PO Box 641946
Omaha, NE 68164
402-905-2794
http://www.nebraskalowvision.com/

Lions Clubs International
https://directory.lionsclubs.org/?language=EN

State Office for National Library Services (NLS)
Nebraska Library Commission

Talking Book and Braille Service
The Atrium
1200 N Street, Suite 120
Lincoln, NE 68508-2023
402-471-4038
http://nlc.nebraska.gov/tbbs/
Serves: Nebraska; braille readers receive service from Utah.

Nevada

State Agency for the Blind and Visually Impaired

Nevada Bureau of Services to the Blind and Visually Impaired
1370 S. Curry Street
Carson City, NV 89703
775-684-4040
http://detr.state.nv.us/rehab/reh_bvi.htm

State Office—VA Visual Impairment Services Team (VIST)

VA Southern Nevada Healthcare System (VASNHS)
3525 W. Cheyanne Avenue
Las Vegas, NV 89032
702-791-9000, x15981

VA Sierra Nevada HCS
1000 Locust Street

Reno, NV 89502
775-326-5715

American Optometric Association
http://www.aoa.org/doctor-locator-search?tab=basic&sso=y

American Academy of Ophthalmology
https://secure.aao.org/aao/find-ophthalmologist

NEI's National Eye Health Education Program
https://nei.nih.gov/nehep

State Organizations and Businesses Providing Low-Vision Support, Products, and Services
Blind Center of Nevada
1001 N. Bruce Street
Las Vegas, NV 89101
702-642-6000
http://www.blindcenter.org

Blindconnect Inc.
6375 W. Charleston Boulevard-WCL200
Las Vegas, NV 89146
702-631-9009
http://blindconnect.org/

Lions Clubs International
https://directory.lionsclubs.org/?language=EN

State Office for National Library Services (NLS)
Nevada Talking Book Services
Nevada State Library, Archives and Public Records
100 N. Stewart Street
Carson City, NV 89701-4285
775-684-3354
http://nsla.nv.gov/Library/Talking_Books/Nevada_Talking_Book_Services/

NEW HAMPSHIRE

State Agency for the Blind and Visually Impaired
New Hampshire Department of Education: Services for Blind and Visually Impaired
21 S. Fruit Street
Walker Building, Suite 20
Concord, NH 03301
603-271-3537
http://education.nh.gov/career/vocational/blind_visu.htm

State Office—VA Visual Impairment Services Team (VIST)
Manchester VAMC
718 Smyth Road

Manchester, NH 03104
603-624-4366, x6475

American Optometric Association
http://www.aoa.org/doctor-locator-search?tab=basic&sso=y

American Academy of Ophthalmology
https://secure.aao.org/aao/find-ophthalmologist

NEI's National Eye Health Education Program
https://nei.nih.gov/nehep

State Organizations and Businesses Providing Low-Vision Support, Products, and Services
New Hampshire Association for the Blind
McGreal Sight Center
25 Walker Street
Concord, NH 03301
603-224-4039
http://www.sightcenter.org

Lions Clubs International
https://directory.lionsclubs.org/?language=EN

State Office for National Library Services (NLS)
New Hampshire State Library

Talking Book Services
117 Pleasant Street
Concord, NH 03301-3852
603-271-3429
http://www.nh.gov/nhsl/talking_books/
Serves: New Hampshire; braille readers receive service from Massachusetts.

New Jersey

State Agency for the Blind and Visually Impaired

New Jersey Commission for the Blind and Visually Impaired
(A Division of the State Department of Human Services)
153 Halsey Street, Sixth Floor
Newark, NJ 07102
973-648-3333
www.cbvi.nj.gov

State Office—VA Visual Impairment Services Team (VIST)

East Orange Campus of the VA New Jersey Health Care System
385 Tremont Avenue
East Orange, NJ 07018
973-676-1000, x1842

American Optometric Association
http://www.aoa.org/doctor-locator-search?tab=basic&sso=y

American Academy of Ophthalmology
https://secure.aao.org/aao/find-ophthalmologist

NEI's National Eye Health Education Program
https://nei.nih.gov/nehep

State Organizations and Businesses Providing Low-Vision Support, Products, and Services
South Jersey Eye Center
400 Chambers Avenue
Camden, NJ 08103
856-365-1811
www.sjeyecenter.org

Vision Loss Alliance
155 Morris Avenue, Suite 2
Denville, NJ 07834
973-627-0055
http://vlanj.org/programs/essential-low-vision/

Lions Clubs International
https://directory.lionsclubs.org/?language=EN

State Office for National Library Services (NLS)
New Jersey State Library Talking Book and Braille Center
2300 Stuyvesant Avenue
Trenton, NJ 08618-3226
609-406-7179
http://www.njstatelib.org/about/contact_us/talking_books_and-braille/
Serves: New Jersey

NEW MEXICO

State Agency for the Blind and Visually Impaired
New Mexico Commission for the Blind
2905 Rodeo Park Drive East
Building 4, Suite 100
Santa Fe, NM 87505
505-476-4479
http://www.cfb.state.nm.us/

State Office—VA Visual Impairment Services Team (VIST)
New Mexico VA Health Care System
1501 San Pedro Drive SE
Albuquerque, NM 87108
505-265-1711, x2774

American Optometric Association
http://www.aoa.org/doctor-locator-search?tab=basic&sso=y

American Academy of Ophthalmology
https://secure.aao.org/aao/find-ophthalmologist

NEI's National Eye Health Education Program
https://nei.nih.gov/nehep

State Organizations and Businesses Providing Low-Vision Support, Products, and Services
NanoPac Inc.
4823 S. Sheridan Road, Suite 302
Tulsa, OK 74145
800-580-6086
http://www.nanopac.com/

New Mexico Technology Assistance Program
625 Silver Street SW
Albuquerque, NM 87102
505-841-4464
http://www.tap.gcd.state.nm.us/

Lions Clubs International
https://directory.lionsclubs.org/?language=EN

State Office for National Library Services (NLS)
New Mexico Library for the Blind and Physically Handicapped
New Mexico State Library
1209 Camino Carlos Rey
Santa Fe, NM 87507-5166
505-476-9770
http://www.nmstatelibrary.org/direct-and-rural-services/lbph
Serves: New Mexico; braille readers receive service from Utah.

NEW YORK

State Agency for the Blind and Visually Impaired
New York State Commission for the Blind
52 Washington Street
Rensselaer, NY 12144
866-871-3000
http://ocfs.ny.gov/main/cb/

State Office—VA Visual Impairment Services Team (VIST)
James J. Peters VAMC—Bronx, NY
130 W. Kingsbridge Road
Bronx, NY 10468
718-584-9000, x1620

VA Western New York Healthcare System at Buffalo
3495 Bailey Avenue
Buffalo, NY 14215
716-862-8782

Canandaigua VAMC
400 Fort Hill Avenue
Canandaigua, NY 14424
585-393-7131

Bath VAMC
76 Veterans Avenue
Bath, NY 14810
607-664-4632

Syracuse VAMC
800 Irving Avenue
Syracuse, NY 13210
315-425-4400, x54010

Albany VAMC
113 Holland Avenue
Albany, NY 12208
518-626-5587

Franklin Delano Roosevelt Campus of the VA Hudson Valley Health Care System (Montrose)

2094 Albany Post Road
Montrose, NY 10548
914-737-4400, x2585

Castle Point Campus of the VA Hudson Valley Health Care System
Route 9D
Castle Point, NY 12511
845-831-2000, x5326

Manhattan Campus of the VA NY Harbor Healthcare System
423 E. Twenty-Third Street
New York, NY 10010
212-686-7500, x3731

Brooklyn Campus of the VA NY Harbor Healthcare System
800 Poly Place
Brooklyn, NY 11209
718-836-6600, x6846

Northport VAMC
79 Middleville Road
Northport, NY 11768
631-261-4400, x2350

American Optometric Association
http://www.aoa.org/doctor-locator-search?tab=basic&sso=y

American Academy of Ophthalmology
https://secure.aao.org/aao/find-ophthalmologist

NEI's National Eye Health Education Program
https://nei.nih.gov/nehep

State Organizations and Businesses Providing Low-Vision Support, Products, and Services
American Foundation for the Blind
Two Penn Plaza, Suite 1102
New York, NY 10121
212-502-7600
http://www.afb.org

Association for the Visually Impaired
260 Old Nyack Turnpike
Spring Valley, NY 10977
845-574-4950
http://avieyes.org/

Central Association for the Blind and Visually Impaired
507 Kent Street
Utica, NY 13501

315-797-2233
http://www.cabvi.org/services/low-vision-care/

Chautauqua Blind Association
510 W. Fifth Street
Jamestown, NY 14701
716-664-6660
http://www.chautauquablind.org/

Olmsted Center for Sight
1170 Main Street
Buffalo, NY 14209
716-882-1025
www.olmstedcenter.org

VISIONS/Services for the Blind and Visually Impaired
500 Greenwich Street, Third Floor
New York, NY 10013-1354
212-625-1616
http://www.visionsvcb.org

Lions Clubs International
https://directory.lionsclubs.org/?language=EN

State Office for National Library Services (NLS)
The New York Public Library
Andrew Heiskell Braille and Talking Book Library

40 W. Twentieth Street
New York, NY 10011-4211
212-206-5400
http://www.nypl.org/locations/heiskell
Serves: New York, Brooklyn (Kings County), Queens, Bronx, Staten Island (Richmond County), Nassau, and Suffolk

New York State Talking Book and Braille Library
Cultural Education Center
222 Madison Avenue
Albany, NY 12230-0001
518-474-5935
http://www.nysl.nysed.gov/tbbl/
Serves: New York State, except New York City and Long Island

Long Island Talking Book Advisory and Outreach Center
Outreach Services
Suffolk Cooperative Library System
627 N. Sunrise Service Road
Bellport, NY 11713-9000
631-286-1600
Serves: Nassau and Suffolk counties

North Carolina

State Agency for the Blind and Visually Impaired

North Carolina Division of Services for the Blind

2601 Mail Service Center
309 Ashe Avenue
Raleigh, NC 27699-2601
919-733-9822
http://www.ncdhhs.gov/dsb/

State Office—VA Visual Impairment Services Team (VIST)

Durham VAMC
508 Fulton Street
Durham, NC 27705
919-286-5235

Fayetteville VAMC
2300 Ramsey Street
Fayetteville, NC 28301
910-488-2120, x5672

Charles George VAMC
1100 Tunnel Road
Asheville, NC 28805
828-298-7911 x5432

Winston-Salem OPC
190 Kimel Park Drive
Winston-Salem, NC 27103
336-768-3296 x1483

Charlotte CBOC
8601 University East Drive
Charlotte, NC 28213
704-597-3500 x7032

American Optometric Association
http://www.aoa.org/doctor-locator-search?tab=basic&sso=y

American Academy of Ophthalmology
https://secure.aao.org/aao/find-ophthalmologist

NEI's National Eye Health Education Program
https://nei.nih.gov/nehep

State Organizations and Businesses Providing Low-Vision Support, Products, and Services
Low Vision Center of Mission Hospitals
240 Sardis Road
Asheville, NC 28806
828-213-4370
http://www.mission-health.org/mission-low-vision.php

North Carolina Memorial Hospital: Low Vision Clinic
Ambulatory Care Center, Second Floor
Mason Farm Road
Chapel Hill, NC 27599

919-966-2061
http://www.med.unc.edu/ophth

Duke Eye Center
2351 Erwin Road
Durham, NC 27705
855-855-6484
https://www.dukemedicine.org/treatments/eye-care

Lions Clubs International
https://directory.lionsclubs.org/?language=EN

State Office for National Library Services (NLS)
North Carolina Library for the Blind and Physically Handicapped
State Library of North Carolina
Department of Natural and Cultural Resources
1841 Capital Boulevard
Raleigh, NC 27604-2188
919-733-4376
http://statelibrary.ncdcr.gov/lbph/
Serves: North Carolina

North Dakota

State Agency for the Blind and Visually Impaired
North Dakota Vision Rehabilitation Services

1237 West Divide Avenue, Suite 1B
Bismarck, ND 58501-1208
701-328-8950
http://www.nd.gov/dhs/dvr/individual/older-blind.html

State Office—VA Visual Impairment Services Team (VIST)
Fargo VAMC
2101 Elm Street
Fargo, ND 58102
701-232-3241, x33056

American Optometric Association
http://www.aoa.org/doctor-locator-search?tab=basic&sso=y

American Academy of Ophthalmology
https://secure.aao.org/aao/find-ophthalmologist

NEI's National Eye Health Education Program
https://nei.nih.gov/nehep

State Organizations and Businesses Providing Low-Vision Support, Products, and Services
North Dakota Assistive
3240-15th Street South, Suite B

Fargo, ND 58104
701-365-4728
http://ndipat.org/vision

Low Vision Products & Training of ND
3801 Memorial Highway, Suite A
Mandad, ND 58554
701-214-4785
http://www.lowvisionnd.com/

Lions Clubs International
https://directory.lionsclubs.org/?language=EN

State Office for National Library Services (NLS)
North Dakota State Library
Talking Book Services
604 E. Boulevard Avenue
Department 250
Bismarck, ND 58505-0800
701-328-1408
http://library.nd.gov/talkingbooks.html
Serves: North Dakota; braille readers receive service from Utah.

Ohio

State Agency for the Blind and Visually Impaired

Opportunities for Ohioans with Disabilities, Bureau of Services for the Visually Impaired and Bureau of Vocational Rehabilitation
150 E. Campus View Boulevard
Columbus, OH 43235
614-438-1200 extension 2 for VR
http://www.ood.ohio.gov/Core-Services/BSVI

State Office—VA Visual Impairment Services Team (VIST)

Chalmers P. Wylie Independent Outpatient Clinic
420 N. James Road
Columbus, OH 43219
614-257-5470

Chillicothe VA Medical Center
17273 State Route 104
Chillicothe, OH 45601
740-773-1141, x6135

Cincinnati VAMC
3200 Vine Street
Cincinnati, OH 45220
937-268-6511, x2176

Louis Stokes VAMC
10701 East Boulevard
Cleveland, OH 44106
216-791-3800, x4240

Youngstown OPC
2031 Belmont Avenue
Youngstown, OH 44505
330-740-9200, x1580

Dayton VAMC
4100 W. Third Street
Dayton, OH 45428
937-268-6511, x3514

American Optometric Association
http://www.aoa.org/doctor-locator-search?tab=basic&sso=y

American Academy of Ophthalmology
https://secure.aao.org/aao/find-ophthalmologist

NEI's National Eye Health Education Program
https://nei.nih.gov/nehep

State Organizations and Businesses Providing Low-Vision Support, Products, and Services

Cincinnati Association for the Blind and Visually Impaired
2045 Gilbert Avenue
Cincinnati, OH 45202-1490
513-221-8558
http://www.cincyblind.org

Cleveland Sight Center
1909 E. 101st Street
Cleveland, OH 44106
216-791-8118
http://www.clevelandsightcenter.org

Judith A. Read Low Vision Services
701 South Main Street
Akron, Ohio 44311-1019
330-762-9755
http://www.udsakron.org/what-we-do/judith-a-read-low-vision-services.aspx

Clovernook Center for the Blind and Visually Impaired, Main Campus
7000 Hamilton Avenue
Cincinnati, OH 45231
513-522-3860
http://www.clovernook.org

Ohio State University: College of Optometry, Low Vision Rehabilitation Service
338 W. Tenth Avenue
Columbus, OH 43210
614-292-1104
http://greatvision.osu.edu/

Philomatheon Society of the Blind
2701 W. Tuscarawas Street
Canton, OH 44708
330-453-9157
http://www.philomatheon.com/

Sight Center of Northwest Ohio: Toledo Society for the Blind
1002 Garden Lake Parkway
Toledo, OH 43614
419-720-3937
http://www.sightcentertoledo.org

Southeast Ohio Sight Center
358 Lincoln Avenue, Unit A
Lancaster, OH 43130
740-687-4785
http://www.orgsites.com/oh/seohiosightcenter/

Lions Clubs International
https://directory.lionsclubs.org/?language=EN

State Office for National Library Services (NLS)
Ohio Library for the Blind and Physically Disabled
Cleveland Public Library
17121 Lake Shore Boulevard
Cleveland, OH 44110-4006
216-623-2911
http://cpl.org/thelibrary/ohio-library-for-the-blind-physically-disabled/
Serves: Ohio

Oklahoma

State Agency for the Blind and Visually Impaired
Oklahoma Department of Rehabilitation Services
3535 NW Fifty-Eighth Street, Suite 500
Oklahoma City, OK 73112
405-951-3400
http://www.okdrs.gov

State Office—VA Visual Impairment Services Team (VIST)
Muskogee VAMC
1011 Honor Heights Drive

Muskogee, OK 74401
918-577-3666

Ernest Childers Tulsa VA. Outpatient Clinic
9322 E. Forty-First Street
Tulsa, OK 74145
918-628-2556

Oklahoma City VAMC
921 NE Thirteenth Street
Oklahoma City, OK 73104
405-456-3915

American Optometric Association
http://www.aoa.org/doctor-locator-search?tab=
basic&sso=y

American Academy of Ophthalmology
https://secure.aao.org/aao/find-ophthalmologist

NEI's National Eye Health Education Program
https://nei.nih.gov/nehep

State Organizations and Businesses Providing Low-Vision Support, Products, and Services
NanoPac Inc.
4823 S. Sheridan Road, Suite 302

Tulsa, OK 74145
800-580-6086
http://www.nanopac.com/

Dean A. McGee Eye Institute
608 Stanton L. Young Boulevard
Oklahoma City, OK 73104
405-271-6060
http://www.dmei.org

Northeastern State University Oklahoma College of Optometry
Northeastern State University
Oklahoma College of Optometry
1001 N. Grand Avenue
Tahlequah, OK 74464
918-444-4090
http://optometry.nsuok.edu/

Lions Clubs International
https://directory.lionsclubs.org/?language=EN

State Office for National Library Services (NLS)
Oklahoma Library for the Blind and Physically Handicapped
300 NE Eighteenth Street

Oklahoma City, OK 73105-3212
405-521-3514
http://www.olbph.org/
Serves: Oklahoma; braille readers receive service from Utah.

OREGON

State Agency for the Blind and Visually Impaired

Oregon Commission for the Blind
535 SE Twelfth Avenue
Portland, OR 97214
971-673-1588
http://www.oregon.gov/blind

State Office—VA Visual Impairment Services Team (VIST)

Portland VAMC
3710 SW US Veterans Hospital Road
Portland, OR 97239
503-402-2986

VA Roseburg Healthcare System
913 NW Garden Valley Boulevard
Roseburg, OR 97470
541-440-1000, x44384

VA Southern Oregon Rehabilitation Center & Clinics
8495 Crater Lake Highway
White City, OR 97503
541-826-2111, x3300

American Optometric Association
http://www.aoa.org/doctor-locator-search?tab=basic&sso=y

American Academy of Ophthalmology
https://secure.aao.org/aao/find-ophthalmologist

NEI's National Eye Health Education Program
https://nei.nih.gov/nehep

State Organizations and Businesses Providing Low-Vision Support, Products, and Services
Devers Memorial Eye Clinic
1040 NW Twenty-Second Avenue
Portland, OR 97210
503-413-8499
http://www.legacyhealth.org/health-services-and-information/health-services/for-adults-a-z/eye-care/for-patients/vision-rehabilitation.aspx

Pacific University College of Optometry
Forest Grove Family Vision Center

2043 College Way
Forest Grove, OR 97116
503-352-2020
http://www.pacificu.edu/optometry/patients/clinics/forestgrove.cfm

Lions Clubs International
https://directory.lionsclubs.org/?language=EN

State Office for National Library Services (NLS)
Oregon Talking Book and Braille Library
Oregon State Library
250 Winter Street NE
Salem, OR 97301-3950
503-378-5389
http://ORTalkingbooks.org
Serves: Oregon; braille readers receive service from Utah.

Pennsylvania

State Agency for the Blind and Visually Impaired
Pennsylvania Department of Labor and Industry, Office of Vocational Rehabilitation, Bureau of Blindness and Visual Services
1521 N. Sixth Street

Harrisburg, PA 17102
717-787-3201
http://www.dli.pa.gov/Individuals/Disability-Services/bbvs/Pages/default.aspx

State Office—VA Visual Impairment Services Team (VIST)

Altoona—James E. Van Zandt VAMC
2907 Pleasant Valley Boulevard
Altoona, PA 16602
814-943-8164, x7407

Butler VAMC
325 New Castle Road
Butler, PA 16001
724-285-2493

Coatesville VAMC
1400 Black Horse Hill Road
Coatesville, PA 19320
610-384-7711, x3929

Erie VAMC
135 E. Thirty-eight Street
Erie, PA 16504
814-860-2927

Lebanon VAMC
1700 S. Lincoln Avenue
Lebanon, PA 17042
717-272-6621, x5507

Philadelphia VAMC
3900 Woodland Avenues
Philadelphia, PA 19104
215-823-5179

VAPHS
HJH Campus
1010 Delafield Road, Building 71, Room 1B107
Pittsburgh, PA 15215
412-822-2176

Wilkes-Barre VAMC
1111 East End Boulevard
Wilkes-Barre, PA 18711
570-824-3521, x7464

American Optometric Association
http://www.aoa.org/doctor-locator-search?tab=basic&sso=y

American Academy of Ophthalmology
https://secure.aao.org/aao/find-ophthalmologist

NEI's National Eye Health Education Program
https://nei.nih.gov/nehep

State Organizations and Businesses Providing Low-Vision Support, Products, and Services
Allegheny Intermediate Unit: Special Education Division, Blind and Visually Impaired Support Program
475 E. Waterfront Drive
Homestead, PA 15120
412-394-5714
http://www.aiu3.net/Level3.aspx?id=1282

Blind and Vision Rehabilitation Services of Pittsburgh
1800 West Street
Homestead, PA 15120-2578
412-368-4400
http://www.pghvis.org

Center for the Blind and Visually Impaired
100 W. Fifteenth Street
Chester, PA 19013
610-874-1476
http://www.cbvi.net

Center for Vision Loss
845 Wyoming Street
Allentown, PA 18103
610-433-6018
http://centerforvisionloss.org

ForSight Vision
1380 Spahn Avenue
York, PA 17403
717-848-1690
http://www.forsight.org

Penn Center for Low Vision Rehabilitation and Research
Scheie Eye Institute, Department of Ophthalmology
University of Pennsylvania Health System
Ralston House, Room 141
3615 Chestnut Street
Philadelphia, PA 19104
215-662-2600
http://www.pennmedicine.org/ophthalmology/patient-care/eye-diseases/low-vision.html

Lions Clubs International
https://directory.lionsclubs.org/?language=EN

State Office for National Library Services (NLS)
Library for the Blind and Physically Handicapped
Free Library of Philadelphia
919 Walnut Street
Philadelphia, PA 19107-0000
215-683-3213
http://www.freelibrary.org/lbph/
Serves: Bradford, Cumberland, Lycoming, Northumberland, Perry, Philadelphia, Snyder, Sullivan, York, and all other counties in eastern Pennsylvania; braille readers in Delaware, all of Pennsylvania, and West Virginia
Library for the Blind and Physically Handicapped
Carnegie Library of Pittsburgh
Leonard C. Staisey Building
4724 Baum Boulevard
Pittsburgh, PA 15213-1389
412-687-2440
http://www.carnegielibrary.org/lbph
Serves: Entire state of Pennsylvania for audio

PUERTO RICO
State Agency for the Blind and Visually Impaired
Puerto Rico Vocational Rehabilitation Administration

Department of Labor and Human Services
PO Box 191118
San Juan, PR 00919-1118
787-729-0160

State Office—VA Visual Impairment Services Team (VIST)
VA Caribbean Healthcare System
10 Casia Street
San Juan, PR 00921
787-641-7582, x31291

VAMC
Paseo Del Veterano #1010
Ponce, PR 00716
(Ponce) 787-812-3030, x44261
(Mayaguez) 787-834-6900, x48047

American Optometric Association
http://www.aoa.org/doctor-locator-search?tab=basic&sso=y

American Academy of Ophthalmology
https://secure.aao.org/aao/find-ophthalmologist

NEI's National Eye Health Education Program
https://nei.nih.gov/nehep

State Organizations and Businesses Providing Low-Vision Support, Products, and Services
Puerto Rico Assistive Technology Program
University of Puerto Rico
FILIUS Institute
Jardin Botanico Sur
1187 Calle Flamboyan
San Juan, PR 00926
787-764-6023
http://www.pratp.upr.edu

Lions Clubs International
https://directory.lionsclubs.org/?language=EN

State Office for National Library Services (NLS)
Puerto Rico Regional Library for the Blind and Physically Handicapped
520 De la Constitución Avenue, Suite 2
San Juan, PR 00901-0000
787-723-2519 or 787-721-7178
Serves: Puerto Rico

Rhode Island

State Agency for the Blind and Visually Impaired

Rhode Island Department of Human Services: Services for the Blind and Visually Impaired
40 Fountain Street
Providence, RI 02903
401-277-2382
http://www.ors.state.ri.us/SBVI.html

State Office—VA Visual Impairment Services Team (VIST)

Providence VAMC
830 Chalkstone Avenue
Providence, RI 02908
401-273-7100, x1554

American Optometric Association

http://www.aoa.org/doctor-locator-search?tab=basic&sso=y

American Academy of Ophthalmology

https://secure.aao.org/aao/find-ophthalmologist

NEI's National Eye Health Education Program

https://nei.nih.gov/nehep

State Organizations and Businesses Providing Low-Vision Support, Products, and Services

IN-SIGHT
43 Jefferson Boulevard, Suite 1
Warwick, RI 02888
401-941-3322
http://www.in-sight.org/index.php/our-solutions/low-vision-clinic

State Office for National Library Services (NLS)

Talking Books Plus
Office of Library and Information Services
One Capitol Hill
Providence, RI 02908-5803
401-574-9310
http://www.olis.ri.gov/tbp/
Serves: Rhode Island; Braille readers served by MA1A. (Perkins Braille and Talking Book Library)

South Carolina

State Agency for the Blind and Visually Impaired

South Carolina Commission for the Blind
1430 Confederate Avenue
Columbia, SC 29201
803-898-8764
http://www.sccb.state.sc.us/

State Office—VA Visual Impairment Services Team (VIST)
Ralph H. Johnson VAMC
109 Bee Street
Charleston, SC 29401
843-789-7575

Wm. Jennings Bryan Dorn VAMC
6439 Garners Ferry Road
Columbia, SC 29209
803-776-4000, x7195

American Optometric Association
http://www.aoa.org/doctor-locator-search?tab=basic&sso=y

American Academy of Ophthalmology
https://secure.aao.org/aao/find-ophthalmologist

NEI's National Eye Health Education Program
https://nei.nih.gov/nehep

State Organizations and Businesses Providing Low-Vision Support, Products, and Services
Feldberg Center for Vision Rehabilitation
Storm Eye Institute
167 Ashley Avenue

MSC 676
Charleston, SC 29425
http://www.muschealth.org/eyes/services/low-vision/index.html
Southern Eye Associates
113 Doctors Drive
Greenville, SC 29605
864-269-3333
https://southern-eye.com/service/low-vision/

Lions Clubs International
https://directory.lionsclubs.org/?language=EN

State Office for National Library Services (NLS)
South Carolina State Library
1500 Senate Street
Columbia, SC 29201
803-734-4611
http://sctalkingbook.org
Serves: South Carolina; braille readers receive service from Utah.

South Dakota

State Agency for the Blind and Visually Impaired
South Dakota Division of Service to the Blind and Visually Impaired

Hillsview Properties Plaza
3800 E. Highway 34, c/o 500 E. Capital
Pierre, SD 57501
605-773-4644
http://dhs.sd.gov/servicetotheblind/default.aspx

State Office—VA Visual Impairment Services Team (VIST)
Sioux Falls VAMC
2501 W. Twenty-Second Street
Sioux Falls, SD 57117
605-336-3230

VA Black Hills Health Care System—Hot Springs Campus
500 N. Fifth Street
Hot Springs, SD 57747
605-745-2000, x92558

American Optometric Association
http://www.aoa.org/doctor-locator-search?tab=basic&sso=y

American Academy of Ophthalmology
https://secure.aao.org/aao/find-ophthalmologist

NEI's National Eye Health Education Program
https://nei.nih.gov/nehep

State Organizations and Businesses Providing Low-Vision Support, Products, and Services

Black Hills Regional Eye Institute
2800 Third Street
Rapid City, SD 57701
605-341-2000
http://www.lasikrapidcity.com/low-vision.htm

Lions Clubs International

https://directory.lionsclubs.org/?language=EN

State Office for National Library Services (NLS)

South Dakota Braille and Talking Book Library
Mercedes Mackay Building
800 Governors Drive
Pierre, SD 57501-2294
605-773-3131
http://library.sd.gov/BTB
Serves: South Dakota; braille readers receive service from Utah.

Tennessee

State Agency for the Blind and Visually Impaired

Tennessee Services for the Blind and Visually Impaired
400 Deaderick Street, Eleventh Floor
Nashville, TN 37248

615-313-4914
http://www.tn.gov/humanservices/topic/blind-visually-impaired-services

State Office—VA Visual Impairment Services Team (VIST)
Veterans Affairs Medical Center
1030 Jefferson Avenue
Memphis, TN 38104
901-523-8990 x15577

Mountain Home VAMC
PO Box 4000
Mountain Home, TN 37684
423-926-1171, x2979

Tennessee Valley Healthcare System, Nashville Campus
1310 Twenty-Fourth Avenue South
Nashville, TN 37212
800-228-4973 x66770

American Optometric Association
http://www.aoa.org/doctor-locator-search?tab=basic&sso=y

American Academy of Ophthalmology
https://secure.aao.org/aao/find-ophthalmologist

NEI's National Eye Health Education Program
https://nei.nih.gov/nehep

State Organizations and Businesses Providing Low-Vision Support, Products, and Services
Eye Center at Southern College of Optometry
1225 Madison Avenue
Memphis, TN 38104
901-722-3250
http://tec.sco.edu/visiontherapyandrehabilitation

Lions Clubs International
https://directory.lionsclubs.org/?language=EN

State Office for National Library Services (NLS)
Tennessee Library for the Blind and Physically Handicapped
Tennessee State Library and Archives
403 Seventh Avenue North
Nashville, TN 37243-1409
615-741-3915
http://sos.tn.gov/tsla/lbph
Serves: Tennessee

Texas

State Agency for the Blind and Visually Impaired

Texas Department of Assistive and Rehabilitative Services: Division for Blind Services
4800 N. Lamar Boulevard, Suite 310
Austin, TX 78756-3178
512-377-0500
http://www.dars.state.tx.us

State Office—VA Visual Impairment Services Team (VIST)

Michael E. DeBakey VAMC
2002 Holcombe Boulevard
Houston, TX 77030
713-791-1414, x25327
713-791-1414, x25398

Amarillo VA Health Care System
6010 Amarillo Boulevard West
Amarillo, TX 79106
806-472-3400, x3553

VA North Texas Health Care System: Dallas VAMC
4500 S. Lancaster Road
Dallas, TX 75216
214-857-2018

South Texas Veterans HCS
7400 Merton Minter Boulevard
San Antonio, TX 78229
210-949-8928
210-949-8929

Harlingen VET Health Care Center
2601 Veterans Drive
Harlingen, TX 78550
956-291-9000, x69235

El Paso VA Health Care System
5001 N. Piedras Street
El Paso, TX 79930
915-564-6102

Central Texas Veterans Health Care System
7901 Metropolis Drive
Austin, TX 78744
512-823-4142

American Optometric Association
http://www.aoa.org/doctor-locator-search?tab=basic&sso=y

American Academy of Ophthalmology
https://secure.aao.org/aao/find-ophthalmologist

NEI's National Eye Health Education Program
https://nei.nih.gov/nehep

State Organizations and Businesses Providing Low-Vision Support, Products, and Services
Texas Department of Assistive and Rehabilitative Services: Criss Cole Rehabilitation Center
4800 N. Lamar Boulevard, CCRC
Austin, TX 78756
512-377-0300
http://www.dars.state.tx.us/dbs/ccrc/index.shtml

Center for Sight Enhancement, Low Vision Rehabilitation
University of Houston
4901 Calhoun Road
Houston, TX 77204
713-743-0799
https://www.opt.uh.edu/patient-care/uei/our-services/low-vision/what-is-low-vision/

Center for Visual Rehabilitation
The Robert Cizik Eye Clinic
Memorial Hermann Medical Plaza
6400 Fannin Street, Eighteenth Floor
Houston, TX 77030
713-559-5269
http://www.cizikeye.org/low-vision-visual-rehabilitation/

Christal Vision
106 Evans Oak Lane
San Antonio, TX 78260
210-666-0700
http://www.christal-vision.com/

Dallas Lighthouse for the Blind
4306 Capitol Avenue
Dallas, TX 75204
214-821-2375
http://www.dallaslighthouse.org/services_seniors.html

East Texas Lighthouse for the Blind | The Lighthouse
411 W. Front Street
Tyler, TX 75702
903-593-3111
http://tylerlighthouse.org/services/low-vision-store/

Lighthouse for the Blind of Fort Worth
912 W. Broadway Avenue
Fort Worth, TX 76104
817-332-3341
http://lighthousefw.org/client-services/#assistive-tech

Lighthouse of Houston
3602 W. Dallas Avenue
Houston, TX 77019-0435

713-527-9561
http://www.houstonlighthouse.org/community-services-center/

Lions Low Vision Center of Texas
Department of Ophthalmology
8403 Floyd Curl Drive
San Antonio, TX 78229
210-567-8600
http://www.uthscsa.edu/patient-care/utmedicine/services/low-vision-services

San Antonio Lighthouse for the Blind
2305 Roosevelt Avenue
San Antonio, TX 78210
210-531-1533
https://www.salighthouse.org/programs/vision-rehabilitation-center/

Lions Clubs International
https://directory.lionsclubs.org/?language=EN

State Office for National Library Services (NLS)
Texas State Library and Archives Commission
Talking Book Program
1201 Brazos Street
Austin, TX 78711-2927

512-463-5458
http://www.texastalkingbooks.org
Serves: Texas

Utah

State Agency for the Blind and Visually Impaired

Utah State Division of Services for the Blind and Visually Impaired (DSBVI)
250 North 1950 West, Suite B
Salt Lake City, UT 84116-7902
801-323-4343
https://www.usor.utah.gov/home-blind-visually-impaired

State Office—VA Visual Impairment Services Team (VIST)

VA Salt Lake City HCS
500 Foothill Drive
Salt Lake City, UT 84148
801-582-1565, x1555

American Optometric Association

http://www.aoa.org/doctor-locator-search?tab=basic&sso=y

American Academy of Ophthalmology
https://secure.aao.org/aao/find-ophthalmologist

NEI's National Eye Health Education Program
https://nei.nih.gov/nehep

State Organizations and Businesses Providing Low-Vision Support, Products, and Services
John A. Moran Eye Center
University of Utah
65 Mario Capecchi Drive
Salt Lake City, UT 84132
801-581-2352
http://healthcare.utah.edu/moran/

Lions Clubs International
https://directory.lionsclubs.org/?language=EN

State Office for National Library Services (NLS)
Utah State Library, Program for the Blind and Disabled
250 North 1950 West, Suite A
Salt Lake City, UT 84116-7904
801-715-6789
http://blindlibrary.utah.gov

VERMONT

State Agency for the Blind and Visually Impaired

Vermont Division for the Blind and Visually Impaired
Agency of Human Services
Weeks IC
103 S. Main Street
Waterbury, VT 05671-2304
802-871-3382
http://www.dbvi.vermont.gov/

State Office—VA Visual Impairment Services Team (VIST)

White River Junction VAMC
215 N. Main Street
White River Junction, VT 05009
802-295-9363, x5347

American Optometric Association

http://www.aoa.org/doctor-locator-search?tab=basic&sso=y

American Academy of Ophthalmology

https://secure.aao.org/aao/find-ophthalmologist

NEI's National Eye Health Education Program

https://nei.nih.gov/nehep

State Organizations and Businesses Providing Low-Vision Support, Products, and Services
Vermont Association for the Blind and Visually Impaired
60 Kimball Avenue
South Burlington, VT 05403
802-863-1358
http://www.vabvi.org/vision-rehabilitation-therapy-page/

Lions Clubs International
https://directory.lionsclubs.org/?language=EN

State Office for National Library Services (NLS)
Vermont Department of Libraries
Special Services Unit
578 Paine Turnpike North
Berlin, VT 05602-9139
802-828-3273 or 802-828-3271
http://libraries.vermont.gov/library_for_the_blind
Serves: Vermont; braille readers receive service from Massachusetts.

VIRGIN ISLANDS

State Agency for the Blind and Visually Impaired
Virgin Islands Department of Human Services
Knut Hansen Complex, Building A

1303 Hospital Ground
St. Thomas, VI 00802
340-774-0930
http://www.dhs.gov.vi/home/index.html

State Office—VA Visual Impairment Services Team (VIST)
VA Caribbean Healthcare System
10 Casia Street
San Juan, PR 00921
787-641-7582

American Optometric Association
http://www.aoa.org/doctor-locator-search?tab=basic&sso=y

American Academy of Ophthalmology
https://secure.aao.org/aao/find-ophthalmologist

NEI's National Eye Health Education Program
https://nei.nih.gov/nehep

State Organizations and Businesses Providing Low-Vision Support, Products, and Services
Laser Vision Institute of the Virgin Islands
St. Thomas, Virgin Islands
Nisky Center, Suite 19B

St. Thomas, VI 00802
340-774-3003
http://www.virgin-eyes.com/

Christiansted, Virgin Islands
79 Peter's Rest
Christiansted, VI 00820
340-778-3003

US Virgin Islands
Community Rehabilitation Facilities
http://www.dhs.gov.vi/disabilities/community_rehab.html

Lions Clubs International
https://directory.lionsclubs.org/?language=EN

State Office for National Library Services (NLS)
Virgin Islands Library for the Visually and Physically Handicapped
3012 Golden Rock
Christiansted, VI 00820-0000
340-718-2250
http://www.virginislandspubliclibraries.org/libraryregional.asp
Serves: US Virgin Islands

Virginia

State Agency for the Blind and Visually Impaired

Virginia Department for the Blind and Vision Impaired
397 Azalea Avenue
Richmond, VA 23227-3600
804-371-3140
http://www.vdbvi.org

State Office—VA Visual Impairment Services Team (VIST)

Hampton VAMC
100 Emancipation Drive
Hampton, VA 23667
757-722-9961, x7070

Hunter Holmes McGuire VAMC
1201 Broad Rock Boulevard
Richmond, VA 23249
804-675-5221

Salem VAMC
1970 Roanoke Boulevard
Salem, VA 24153
540-982-2463, x3356

American Optometric Association
http://www.aoa.org/doctor-locator-search?tab=basic&sso=y

American Academy of Ophthalmology
https://secure.aao.org/aao/find-ophthalmologist

NEI's National Eye Health Education Program
https://nei.nih.gov/nehep

State Organizations and Businesses Providing Low-Vision Support, Products, and Services
Aniridia Foundation International
c/o University of Virginia Department of Ophthalmology
PO Box 800715
Charlottesville, VA 22908-0715
434-243-3357
http://www.make-a-miracle.org

Virginia Rehabilitation Center for the Blind and Vision Impaired
401 Azalea Avenue
Richmond, VA 23227
804-371-3151
http://www.vrcbvi.org

Vision Council of America/The Vision Council
225 Reinekers Lane, Suite 700
Alexandria, VA 22314
703-548-4560
www.thevisioncouncil.org

Lions Clubs International
https://directory.lionsclubs.org/?language=EN

State Office for National Library Services (NLS)
Virginia Library and Resource Center
Virginia Department for the Blind and Vision Impaired
395 Azalea Avenue
Richmond, VA 23227-3633
804-371-3661, ext. 135
http://www.vdbvi.org/library_resourcecenter.htm
Serves: Virginia

Alexandria Library-Beatley Central
Talking Book Service
5005 Duke Street
Alexandria, VA 22304-2903
703-746-1760 or 703-746-1762
https://alexlibraryva.org/client/en_US/home
Serves: City of Alexandria

Talking Book Service
Arlington Public Library
1015 N. Quincy Street
Arlington, VA 22201-4603
703-228-6333
http://library.arlingtonva.us/services/special-accommodations/
Serves: Arlington County

Access Services
Fairfax County Public Library
12000 Government Center Parkway, Suite 123
Fairfax, VA 22035-0012
703-324-8380
http://www.fairfaxcounty.gov/library/branches/as/default.htm
Serves: Fairfax County; cities of Fairfax and Falls Church

Roanoke Public Library
Talking Book Services
2607 Salem Turnpike NW
Roanoke, VA 24017-5397
540-853-2648
http://www.roanokegov.com/library/talking.html
Serves: Alleghany, Botetourt, Craig, and Roanoke counties; cities of Clifton Forge, Covington, Roanoke, and Salem

Bayside and Special Services Library, Department of Public Libraries
936 Independence Boulevard
Virginia Beach, VA 23455-0000
757-385-2684
http://www.vbgov.com/government/departments/libraries/Using-the-Library/Pages/Disability-Services.aspx
Serves: Virginia Beach

Talking Book Center
Staunton Public Library
1 Churchville Avenue
Staunton, VA 24401-0000
540-885-6215
http://www.talkingbookcenter.org
Serves: Augusta, Bath, Highland, and Rockbridge counties and the cities of Buena Vista, Lexington, Staunton, and Waynesboro

Fredericksburg Area Subregional Library
Central Rappahannock Regional Library
1201 Caroline Street
Fredericksburg, VA 22401-0000
540-372-1144 extension 234
http://www.librarypoint.org/talking_books

Serves: Fredericksburg, Prince William, Spotsylvania, Stafford, King George, Caroline, Westmoreland, and Orange counties

Washington

State Agency for the Blind and Visually Impaired

Washington State Department of Services for the Blind
4565 Seventh Avenue SE
Lacey, WA 98504-0933
360-725-3830
http://www.dsb.wa.gov/

State Office—VA Visual Impairment Services Team (VIST)

VA Puget Sound HCS 1660
S. Columbian Way
Seattle, WA 98108
206-764-2758

Spokane VAMC
4815 N. Assembly Street
Spokane, WA 99205
509-434-7670

Jonathan M. Wainwright Memorial VAMC
77 Wainwright Drive
Walla Walla, WA 99362
509-525-5200, x26255

VA Puget Sound HCS
1660 S. Columbian Way
Seattle, WA 98108
253-583-1287

American Optometric Association
http://www.aoa.org/doctor-locator-search?tab=basic&sso=y

American Academy of Ophthalmology
https://secure.aao.org/aao/find-ophthalmologist

NEI's National Eye Health Education Program
https://nei.nih.gov/nehep

State Organizations and Businesses Providing Low-Vision Support, Products, and Services
Lilac Services for the Blind
1212 N. Howard Street
Spokane, WA 99201
509-328-9116
http://www.lilacblind.org

SightConnection
9709 Third Avenue NE, Suite 100
Seattle, WA 98115-2027
206-525-5556
http://www.sightconnection.org

Lions Clubs International
https://directory.lionsclubs.org/?language=EN

State Office for National Library Services (NLS)
Washington Talking Book & Braille Library
2021 Ninth Avenue
Seattle, WA 98121-2783
206-615-0400
http://www.wtbbl.org
Serves: Washington

West Virginia

State Agency for the Blind and Visually Impaired
West Virginia Division of Rehabilitation Services
107 Capitol Street
Charleston, WV 25301-2609
304-356-2060
http://www.wvdrs.org

State Office—VA Visual Impairment Services Team (VIST)

Beckley VAMC
200 Veterans Avenue
Beckley, WV 25801
304-255-2121, x4223

Louis A. Johnson VAMC
One Medical Center Drive
Clarksburg, WV 26301
304-623-3461, x3695

Huntington VAMC
1540 Spring Valley Drive
Huntington, WV 25704
304-429-6741, x2847

Martinsburg VAMC
510 Butler Avenue
Martinsburg, WV 25405
304-263-0811

American Optometric Association

http://www.aoa.org/doctor-locator-search?tab=basic&sso=y

American Academy of Ophthalmology
https://secure.aao.org/aao/find-ophthalmologist

NEI's National Eye Health Education Program
https://nei.nih.gov/nehep

State Organizations and Businesses Providing Low-Vision Support, Products, and Services
AFB Tech
1000 Fifth Avenue, Suite 350
Huntington, WV 25701
304-523-8651
http://www.afb.org/info/living-with-vision-loss/1

WVU Eye Institute
1 Medical Center Drive
Morgantown, WV 26506
304-598-4820
http://wvumedicine.org/hospitals-and-institutes/eye-institute/

Lions Clubs International
https://directory.lionsclubs.org/?language=EN

State Office for National Library Services (NLS)
West Virginia Library Commission-Special Services Libraries

Blind and Physically Handicapped Services
Cultural Center
1900 Kanawha Boulevard East
Charleston, WV 25305-0620
304-558-4061
http://www.librarycommission.wv.gov/services/special-services/Pages/default.aspx
Serves: West Virginia; braille readers receive service from Philadelphia.

Services for the Blind and Physically Handicapped
Cabell County Public Library
455 Ninth Street Plaza
Huntington, WV 25701-0000
304-528-5700
http://cabell.lib.wv.us/pages/talkbook.htm
Serves: Cabell, Mason, Mingo, Putnam, and Wayne counties

Services for the Blind and Physically Handicapped
Parkersburg and Wood County Public Library
3100 Emerson Avenue
Parkersburg, WV 26104-2414
304-420-4587
Serves: Calhoun, Jackson, Pleasants, Ritchie, Roane, Tyler, Wirt, and Wood counties

West Virginia School for the Blind
Library
301 E. Main Street
Romney, WV 26757-0000
304-822-4894 or 304-822-6656
Serves: Berkeley, Grant, Hampshire, Hardy, Jefferson, Mineral, Morgan, and Pendleton counties

Wisconsin

State Agency for the Blind and Visually Impaired
Wisconsin Department of Workforce Development: Division of Vocational Rehabilitation
201 E. Washington Avenue
Madison, WI 53707-7852
608-261-0050
http://dwd.wisconsin.gov/dvr/

State Office—VA Visual Impairment Services Team (VIST)
William S. Middleton Memorial Veterans Hospital
2500 Overlook Terrace
Madison, WI 53705
608-256-1901, x11960

Tomah VAMC
500 E. Veterans Street

Tomah, WI 54660
608-372-3971, 66440

Clement J. Zablocki Veterans Affairs Medical Center
5000 W. National Avenue
Milwaukee, WI 53295
414-384-2000, x41832

American Optometric Association
http://www.aoa.org/doctor-locator-search?tab=basic&sso=y

American Academy of Ophthalmology
https://secure.aao.org/aao/find-ophthalmologist

NEI's National Eye Health Education Program
https://nei.nih.gov/nehep

State Organizations and Businesses Providing Low-Vision Support, Products, and Services
Low Vision Rehabilitation Service: University Station Clinics
2880 University Avenue
Madison, WI 53705
608-263-7171
http://www.uwhealth.org/eyecare/low-vision-service/10783

Lions Clubs International
https://directory.lionsclubs.org/?language=EN

State Office for National Library Services (NLS)
Wisconsin Talking Book and Braille Library
813 W. Wells Street
Milwaukee, WI 53233-1436
414-286-3045
http://dpi.wi.gov/talkingbooks
Serves: Wisconsin; braille readers receive service from Utah.

WYOMING

State Agency for the Blind and Visually Impaired
Wyoming Division of Vocational Rehabilitation
614 S. Greeley Highway
Cheyenne, WY 82002
307-777-7389
http://wyomingworkforce.org/workers/vr/

State Office—VA Visual Impairment Services Team (VIST)
Cheyenne VA Medical
2360 E. Pershing Boulevard
Cheyenne, WY 82001
307-433-3607

Sheridan VAMC
1898 Fort Road
Sheridan, WY 82801
307-675-3307

American Optometric Association
http://www.aoa.org/doctor-locator-search?tab=basic&sso=y

American Academy of Ophthalmology
https://secure.aao.org/aao/find-ophthalmologist

NEI's National Eye Health Education Program
https://nei.nih.gov/nehep

State Organizations and Businesses Providing Low-Vision Support, Products, and Services
Casper Senior Center
1831 E. Fourth Street
Casper, WY 82601
307-234-3980
https://wyomingmedicalcenter.org/support/low-vision

Lions Clubs International
https://directory.lionsclubs.org/?language=EN

National Library Services (NLS)
Wyoming served by Utah
Utah State Library Division
Program for the Blind and Disabled
250 North 1950 West, Suite A
Salt Lake City, UT 84116-7901
801-715-6789
Website: http://blindlibrary.utah.gov/
Serves: Utah, Alaska, Wyoming; braille readers in Alabama, Arizona, Connecticut, Georgia, Idaho, Illinois, Kansas, Louisiana, Mississippi, Montana, Nebraska, Nevada, New Mexico, North Dakota, Oklahoma, Oregon, South Carolina, South Dakota, and Wisconsin

ABOUT THE AUTHOR

PATRICK J. FISCHER BELIEVES THAT technology is the best way to improve the lives of the deaf, blind, and other disabled individuals. When he first entered the computer industry as a technician, he began volunteering to help disabled individuals learn how to use technology.

As Fischer moved through several different jobs in the industry, he continued to help the disabled community. Through his company, eventually called Vision Helpers, he began dedicating his career to helping people with blindness or low vision. In 2002, he opened his first showroom in Omaha, Nebraska, which sold low-vision products. He expanded to another showroom in Des Moines, Iowa.

Fischer has since closed the showrooms and now works directly with individuals, businesses, and doctors to help those in need.

www.ingramcontent.com/pod-product-compliance
Lightning Source LLC
Chambersburg PA
CBHW060847280326
41934CB00007B/945

* 9 7 8 0 6 9 2 8 3 9 1 5 7 *